PROMOTING HEALTH
POLITICS AND PRACTICE

**Edited by
Lee Adams
Mary Amos
James Munro**

SAGE Publications
London • Thousand Oaks • New Delhi

SAGE Publications Ltd
6 Bonhill Street
London EC2A 4PU

SAGE Publications Inc
2455 Teller Road
Thousand Oaks, California 91320

SAGE Publications India Pvt Ltd
32, M-Block Market
Greater Kailash – 1
New Delhi 110 048

British Library Cataloguing in Publication Data
A catalogue record for this book is available from
the British Library

ISBN 0 7619 6833 4
ISBN 0 7619 6834 2 (pbk)

Library of Congress Control Number: 2001135941

Typeset by M Rules
Printed in Great Britain by The Cromwell Press Ltd,
Trowbridge, Wiltshire

CONTENTS

To Godfrey William French, my beloved father who died at 38 years.
(Lee Adams)

For Zeke, Jasmine and Toby, my grandchildren, in the hope that they grow up in healthy communities.
(Mary Amos)

To Mum and Dad, with thanks.
(James Munro)

FOREWORD

Whenever politicians stand back and ask what needs to be done to improve the nation's health, each incoming health minister is struck anew by a simple fact well known to all health practitioners: prevention is better and cheaper than cure. The building of sewers did more in history and does more now in the Third World than the building of high tech hospitals, with more health gain and better value for every pound spent. The most cursory glance at the statistics shows every new health minister that poverty is what drags down NHS outcome figures more than anything else. Excess infant deaths, lung cancer, obesity, heart disease, early death and high child accident rates are all the direct results of a poor and poorly educated population. Even Conservative health ministers admitted this was the undeniable truth.

But once ensconced at the controls of the NHS, the daily rapacious demands of the existing health system sweep all before it. The press, patients and voters demand more beds, shorter waiting lists, more high tech operations and more expensive drugs: each may offer a proven health improvement for the patient, but a relatively small one for the money spent. Trying to wrench money out of the acute sector and spend it instead in the community has confounded ministers of all parties, over many years. After all, even now it remains almost impossible to stop very expensive NHS acute beds being 'blocked' by elderly patients for lack of finding them a care home place in the community, even though it is in everyone's interests to get the patient moved. So consider how much more difficult it is to move sizeable sums away from the acute sector and into community-oriented health promotion and disease prevention programmes.

Labour's solution has been to try to do both. In recent high spending years it has been possible to pledge larger than ever sums to the NHS, and at the same time to direct more money towards alleviating poverty than any government since Attlee. Tony Blair has personally made two key pledges: to match average EU spending levels on health by 2006, and to abolish – yes, abolish – all child poverty by 2020. Both of these will be phenomenally difficult to achieve. At least he did not make Bevan's mistake at the founding of the NHS and assume that higher spending on poverty and health in the short run must lead to less demand eventually, since a healthier and better-off population should need less health care. The history of the past 50 years shows, alas, that the richer and healthier the population grows, the greater the demands become for acute health services too – a puzzling and irritating fact. Those in greatest need tend to be not only poor but also patient and passive, while the more affluent become less patient and more demanding on services.

Within the health service itself, under Labour there has been virtually no serious shift of resources from treatment to prevention. Health Action Zones, designed to nurture prevention schemes in poor areas, are a very small add-on. The post of Public Health Minister has actually been demoted a rung since Tessa Jowell was first appointed. Instead, the real initiatives likely to produce a long-term health gain have come from the Treasury, where Chancellor Gordon Brown's best monument so far has been to direct most available funds towards the poorest. As a result of the Working Families Tax Credit, Child Tax Credit, much higher Child Benefit and a 70 per cent rise in Income Support for children of unemployed parents, the poorest two deciles were some 10 per cent better off by the 2001 election, while the top decile was just a shade worse off as a result of tax and benefit changes. The New Deal for Communities and other regeneration schemes, alongside programmes such as Sure Start and Early Excellence Centres, are attempting to head off disadvantage from the cradle.

But at the same time the divide between richest and poorest still grew in Labour's first term, as it always does in boom times when incomes at the top soar away. Around the world the countries with the sharpest rich–poor gap are the ones with the worst health outcomes. There will come a time when the Labour government will have to admit that it matters – but they have not done so yet. Channelling available extra resources towards the poorest may simply not be enough to meet both the Prime Minister's tough targets, without redistribution from the top as well.

In this wide-ranging book, its authors take a radical look at what public health and health promotion should mean in the broadest social and political context. Too often, narrow definitions of health promotion have resulted in nothing more than exhorting the poor not to smoke or eat fried Mars bars. Here, the real causes and effects of social exclusion are analysed, with new ideas of what social inclusion could and should mean for health and well-being. Everything from the importance of public services and the sense of ownership of those services, to protecting the ecosystem, impacts on public health. Many of the ideas here broadly run with the grain of much thinking among ministers but this should act as a sharp reminder that the Prime Minister's goals are unlikely to be met on the government's present political trajectory.

Polly Toynbee
The Guardian
August 2001

NOTES ON CONTRIBUTORS

Lee Adams has worked in health promotion in the NHS for 26 years, currently as director of the Wakefield health action zone and visiting professor of public health at Sheffield Hallam University. She is also a member of the management boards of the Centre for Public Services and of Public Arts.

Pete Alcock is professor of social policy and administration and head of the Department of Social Policy and Social Work at the University of Birmingham. He is the author of *Social Policy in Britain* and *Understanding Poverty* (both Palgrave) and a number of other books and articles in the social policy field.

Mary Amos is co-ordinator of healthy city work at Portsmouth City Council. She worked in health education and promotion in the NHS for 15 years, and more recently directed the masters course in health promotion at Sheffield Hallam University.

Marian Barnes is reader and director of social research in the Department of Social Policy and Social Work, University of Birmingham. She has a particular interest in collective action among users/survivors of mental health services, older people and other service users.

Alan Beattie has been involved in health education and public health for 25 years, in academic and community settings, and is currently professor of health promotion at St Martin's College Lancaster.

Simon Bullock works as a researcher for Friends of the Earth, on the links between environmental and social issues.

Fiona Campbell is co-ordinator of the Democratic Health Network at the Local Government Information Unit and a member of Oxfam's governing body. She is interested in the role of local government in reducing health inequalities and in issues of democracy and accountability in health under globalization.

Martin Caraher is reader in food and social policy in the Centre for Food Policy at Thames Valley University. He has research interests in the role of community groups in food policy, health promotion in prisons, and the development of public health capacity among professions allied to medicine.

Frances Cunning is director of social and community development at Sheffield health authority.

Maria Duggan is an independent research and policy analyst in public health, and was previously director of policy at the Association for Public Health. She has published widely on health inequalities.

Judith Emanuel is a lecturer in education for primary health care at the University of Manchester, and currently runs a masters programme in Zambia.

Jeff French is director of policy and planning at the Health Development Agency, having worked in the health development field for over twenty years. He has a long-standing interest in the history of public health and health promotion.

Mark Gamsu is Sheffield Healthy City co-ordinator. Previously working with the public sector tenants' movement in London, he has worked in Sheffield for 12 years, as a trainer, housing service manager and social services planner.

Lorraine Gradwell is chief executive of Breakthrough UK, and a deputy chair of the Greater Manchester Coalition of Disabled People. She has a long history of involvement in the disabled peoples' movement, and worked for a spell as co-ordinator of 'Healthy Manchester 2000'.

Sue Greig is Health Improvement Manager for South East Sheffield Primary Care Trust (from November 2001 Senior Lecturer Public Health, Sheffield Hallam University). She is interested in practice which connects tackling health inequalities with sustainable development.

Maddy Halliday is currently Director Scotland and UK development for the Mental Health Foundation and is also Scottish chair of the UK Public Health Association. She gained extensive experience of Health For All initiatives as co-ordinator of Glasgow Healthy City Partnership and Healthy Sheffield.

Deborah Harkins is a public health specialist at Wigan and Bolton Health Authority.

Sue Laughlin is currently Women's Health Coordinator with Greater Glasgow Health Board where she has responsibility for supporting the implementation of the Glasgow Women's Health Policy as it applies to the health service in Glasgow. She is also the co-ordinator of the Glasgow WHO Collaborating Centre for Women's Health.

James Munro is a health services researcher at the Medical Care Research Unit, Sheffield University, and founder editor of *Health Matters* magazine, an independent quarterly on health care and public health policy issues.

Neil Parry is project worker for Sheffield East End Quality Of Life Initiative interested in sustainable community development.

James Petts worked in agriculture and the food industry for over ten years in areas of production, distribution, manufacturing and retail. Since joining Sustain, he has been working on a variety of projects in the areas of urban agriculture, food strategy, local food initiatives, and food poverty.

Geof Rayner is currently chair of the UK Public Health Association and visiting fellow at the centre for food policy, Thames Valley University. He has previously worked for a variety of organizations, including the NHS, local authorities, universities in Britain and America, and WHO.

Hilary Russell is deputy director of the European Institute for Urban Affairs at Liverpool John Moores University. She has extensive experience of evaluating partnership approaches to regeneration and has a special interest in community participation.

Eurig Scandrett has worked in ecological research and adult and community education. He is currently head of community action at Friends of the Earth Scotland, and associate lecturer in environmental policy with the Open University.

Charles Secrett is one of Britain's leading environmentalists. He is executive director of Friends of the Earth and has written extensively on a wide range of environmental issues.

Martine Standish currently works in social and community development in public health at Sheffield health authority, and comes from a background in voluntary sector and social work.

Melissa Stead is senior research officer at Sheffield Hallam University.

Ruth Sutherland is director of the Community Development and Health Network for Northern Ireland. She has worked in and alongside health and social services in both statutory and voluntary/community sector roles for over twenty years.

Charles Webster is a fellow of All Souls College, Oxford. He writes on the history of health care in the twentieth century.

Dexter Whitfield is founder of the Centre for Public Services, which has worked for almost 30 years with public bodies, trade unions and community organizations to develop strategies for improving public services and the welfare state. His latest book is *Public Services or Corporate Welfare: Rethinking the Nation State in the Global Economy* (Pluto, 2001).

INTRODUCTION

This book is about improving people's health, though that might not appear obvious from the Contents pages. Unlike many books on promoting health, we start from the belief that health and illness are not primarily the result of individual choices or a genetic lottery, but of the social structures and economic interests which surround us. We also take the view that the health of each of us is intimately related to the health of all of us. Promoting public health, for us, therefore goes beyond encouraging 'healthy lifestyles', improving health care services or developing 'healthy partnerships' between different organizations, important though these may be. Fundamentally, we believe that the job of securing health for all must involve us in encouraging social changes which lead us to ways of living which are sustainable, equitable and socially just.

A starting position like this might make for a book full of worthy, but impractical, ideas. We hope we have avoided this. Throughout the book, we have tried to blend theory with down-to-earth practice: each chapter introduces a major theme, and is followed by three contributions which either explore a policy issue in greater depth, or present a case study of work which has attempted to put theory into practice – though not necessarily perfectly. In this way, we aim to explore both what *should* be done, and what *can* be done, to improve health.

Our choice of the major themes explored in the book – sustainable development, community development, inequality, regeneration and public services – reflects our understanding of what is really important to improving public health. Yet our frustration, as both practitioners and academics, is that mainstream health policy debate has so far ignored issues of environmental quality, social justice and economic power in favour of constantly calling on individuals – particularly the poorest – to change their 'lifestyle'. This is not a new situation, of course. We agree with Sir George Gregory, who noted in *The Lancet* in 1843: 'The greatest foe to health and long life is poverty. Not only do all epidemic visitations fall with tenfold severity upon the poorest classes of society, but all descriptions of disease find in them their chief victim.' It is about time that this observation was taken seriously by policy-makers and public health specialists. Yet, at the local level, valuable public health expertise is almost completely taken up with running health services rather than working for local and national policies which address poverty.

Since Gregory's time there have, of course, been many social changes which have been intended to improve matters, such as progressive tax and benefit policies, welfare services and health care. But economic inequalities between countries have widened steadily over the past 200 years, and within many countries – most notably the UK and the USA – over the past 20 years, and continue to widen even now; for the first time in history human activity threatens to destroy the global ecosystem on which all life depends; and the size and power of global corporate interests have become so great that many of the world's biggest economies are not nations, but companies. Such changes pose fundamental threats to everyone's health, though the costs, as usual, will fall first on the poorest.

Although resignation, cynicism or despair are understandable responses to this situation, the contributors to this book have tried to show that other responses are also possible. In the chapters and case studies, many examples are presented of activity which attempts, sometimes successfully, to protect and promote health at local and national levels. Much talk in current policy debates is of 'partnership', particularly between the public and private sectors, as if fundamental conflicts of interest can be resolved simply through discussion. We take the view that those with power never give it up voluntarily, and that the pursuit of commercial interest is hardly ever altered by arguments about morality or sustainability. The major steps forward in public health over the past two centuries have come about not through partnership but through grass-roots movements of those who stood to gain – or lose – the most. The promotion of public health will inevitably demand that we enter into conflict with those who, in pursuing their own interests, harm the health of many others.

If you accept, as we do, that the promotion of health is fundamentally a political matter, then the task of promoting better health for all becomes a matter of political strategy and immediately we are faced with a range of dilemmas familiar to all who, over the course of history, have tried to change the world for the better. In a rapidly globalizing world, how far is it worth devoting our energies to local projects? Yet how can we engage with global agendas which make us feel powerless in their enormity? How far can we get with community development and other 'bottom-up' approaches in the face of limits – legal, fiscal, environmental – forcefully imposed from the top down? But how can we ignore the demands of local voices? Should we concentrate on single tangible issues which will engage active participation, such as housing, transport or childcare, or attempt to address the multi-dimensional nature of health and inequality through broader action for social justice?

One of the key challenges facing public health promoters is the way that health, once understood in its social and political context, loses any boundaries it may have had when conceived only within a medical setting. Everything is relevant to health. Everything is a health issue. Though this may be true, and feel like a liberating realization, it is also a trap. Not everything can be thought about, or acted on, at the same time. Inevitably, health promoters must prioritize and focus their efforts if they are not to become exhausted and ineffective.

If there are dilemmas about what health promoters should do, there are also dilemmas about who they should be. If improving health is a political project, why should it be run by competing professionalized groups? How important is technical knowledge or specialist training? And if health is a matter of good housing, employment, environment, and so on, why do we split 'health promotion' and 'public health' professionals off into a separate sphere of policy and practice away from these other groups? Furthermore, the fact that most public health and health promotion practitioners work for the state creates immediate and practical limits to the arguments which can be put forward and the practical approaches which can be taken. Employees of the state must not pursue 'political' activities, however that term is understood, and are not supposed to question the policies of their employer. The result is that there are things which everyone knows, yet nobody can say. Instead we busy ourselves with whatever the current 'public health strategy' demands. Surprisingly, however, as some of the contributors to this book relate, there is scope in many places for much greater boldness in advocating approaches which directly address inequalities of power and resources.

One feature of working for the NHS, in particular, is the astonishing organizational amnesia which seems to follow in the wake of the succession of strategies and priorities passed down through the service. A good sense of history is an important antidote to such forgetfulness, and may help us avoid going around in circles. The first chapter of this book therefore attempts to set the scene with a historical overview of 'public health' and 'health promotion' efforts in Britain over the past 200 years. The chapters which follow this discuss the difficulties of creating a mass public health movement and present case studies of healthy city work and health promotion work in the NHS.

Our environment – in both a local and a global sense – is fundamental to maintaining health, and Chapter 2 explores the central issue of sustainability in human activity and how this relates to health. Grouped with this are chapters on national food policy, local transport policy and activism in support of environmental justice.

Chapter 3 and the related chapters consider issues of community development and user participation in services. This chapter explores in depth the dilemmas inherent in community development approaches, and the differing ideologies of community development and their political implications. The related chapters present case studies of community development work in two very different settings, and an exploration of user participation issues.

Those working in health care and public health settings have always understood, in a very practical way, the effects of inequality and discrimination on health, and 'social inclusion' has recently become a topic of mainstream political discourse. Chapter 4 offers a summary of available evidence on the relationships between health and inequality. This is followed by a related chapter critically assessing the potential of anti-poverty strategies, a case study of a strategic approach to women's health, and an examination of issues of disability and health.

Currently, much of the activity funded through or linked with regeneration schemes includes health promoting work, either explicitly or implicitly. Whether urban or rural, regeneration schemes usually aim to boost the local economy, reduce social exclusion and enhance the local environment. In Chapter 5 the relationship between regeneration policy and public health is explored, with subsequent chapters on local food initiatives, and case studies of a health action zone and a regeneration programme.

The importance of equitable, accessible and effective public services to health is discussed in Chapter 6. Currently there is much interest internationally in restructuring public services in ways which introduce market-like incentives, and in some cases outright privatization of services. The debate over the importance of public ownership is likely to intensify as changes in world trade rules increase the pressure on governments to open their services to marketization. Related chapters discuss the centrality of education to improving health, the much neglected role of local government and a case study of benefits advice in a primary care setting.

Though the various sections of the book can be read independently and in any order, we also hope that you will want to read it all, since the themes we have chosen are all inter-connected, and you may find new ideas and insights for your own work through approaching it from unfamiliar territory. We have tried to avoid jargon, though inevitably one person's jargon is another's everyday language, so we are unlikely to have entirely succeeded. Nonetheless, we hope you will find the arguments presented here interesting and accessible. While we have covered a lot of ground, given the lack of boundaries around public health, we have of course been unable to cover everything of importance, so please forgive us if your own particular area of interest is not included here. As well as analysing and reflecting on existing work, we hope to inspire new enthusiasm and new ideas for health promoting work. Only you will know whether we have succeeded.

Lee Adams
Mary Amos
James Munro
Sheffield and Portsmouth
July 2001

1

THE CYCLE OF CONFLICT: THE HISTORY OF THE PUBLIC HEALTH AND HEALTH PROMOTION MOVEMENTS

Charles Webster and Jeff French

Although the immediate sources of both health promotion and the 'New Public Health' are located in the 1970s, many of the ideas associated with these movements have much deeper roots. This short review sets the development of health promotion and the 'New Public Health' in a wider historical framework. Although we are concerned mainly with the UK, the key features are common to many other national contexts. Most histories of the development of public health, and more recently of health promotion, fail to acknowledge that while methods and motivations may vary, co-ordinated community action to ensure a better life is as old as civilization and remains a feature of every community today. In histories of public health there has been a tendency to assume that concern for better health as a prerequisite for better life is a relatively new, medically led and Eurocentric concept. This assumption is symptomatic of a historic interpretation that seeks to medicalize what has been, and remains, a complex and contested social phenomenon. What is required is a reassessment of the development of public health and health promotion that takes account of the social conflict inherent in these movements. In doing so, it should not be taken as self-evident that we have necessarily built up a sophisticated and objective understanding of the contribution of public health and health promotion to better health. Finally, it is also necessary to bear in mind the fundamental purposes of health promotion and public health, and the extent to which they represent different conceptions of the aspiration to health.

The phrase 'public health' as currently used embodies many of the confusions, vested interests and singular interpretations that have resulted from a simplistic interpretation of its historical development. It could even be argued that the term public health is often used in a spirit of what might be described as conspiratorial confusion – a point made by Alan Milburn as UK Secretary of State for Health:

> 'Public health' understood as the epidemiological analysis of the patterns and causes of population health and ill health gets confused with 'public health' understood as population-level health promotion, which in turn gets confused with 'public health' understood as public health professionals

trained in medicine. So by series of definitional sleights of hand, the argument runs that the health of the population should be mainly improved by population-level health promotion and prevention, which in turn is best delivered, or at least overseen and managed, by medical consultants in public health. The time has come to abandon this lazy thinking and occupational protectionism. (Milburn, 2000)

The minister's evident frustration testifies to the current confusion over definitions of purpose and territorial responsibility among health professionals. Implicit in the above quotation, and most other current discussions of public health, are elements of a definition that have, in fact, been in widespread use over the past 75 years. The goals of public health are usually stated to be preventing disease and promoting health, and the mechanism for realizing these objectives to be organized interventions directed at particular groups or the community as a whole. Clearly, therefore, public health has always been associated in some way with health promotion. While this dual identity has been a source of strength, as noted below, it has also proved to be an effective source of friction. Even before the terms public health and health promotion came into use, dilemmas in defining the objectives of such interventions were apparent. In Britain the first public health manifesto was issued on 25 January 1796, in response to the social upheavals associated with the industrial revolution. This remarkable 'Heads of Resolutions for the consideration of the Board of Health' in Manchester resisted the invitation to censure the labouring people for their moral delinquency; instead, it called for their protection through state intervention involving 'a system of laws for the wise, humane, and equal government' of working conditions (Maltby, 1918: 121–2). Looking forward to the thinking of a much later date, the Manchester manifesto firmly located the root causes of ill health in the prevailing economic system. Although this episode demonstrates that general social activism and a strong liberation philosophy predate modern conceptions of public health, in the event such movements failed to bring about widespread improvements in health, owing to the absolute dominance of forces of economic production.

During the 1840s the early public health movement predominantly focused on sanitary conditions, motivated by a desire to reduce Poor Law support and promote economic efficiency. However, at the same time an alternative perspective which saw patterns of disease as a reflection of social conflict was being put forward by writers such as Friedrich Engels. In *The Condition of the Working Class in England*, in 1844, Engels (1973) cited the mode of economic production as the principal cause of ill health. His justification for public health intervention was one based on notions of social justice rather than efficiency of production.

Most histories of public health label this supposed start of the modern public health movement in the 1840s as the *sanitation phase*, a period characterized by adoption of a medical perspective and concentration on environmental issues such as housing, working conditions, the supply of clean water and the safe disposal of waste. Under the supervision of the newly-invented Medical Officers of Health (MOH), the sanitarians focused on improving the health of working people by bringing about changes in their conditions of everyday living. The motivating forces of this early public health movement were both economic advantage and, to a lesser extent, the maintenance of social cohesion between the working poor and the middle and upper classes.

A more critical perspective is provided by Turshen (1989), who suggests that attempts by some historians to portray public health doctors as the health champions of working people are misplaced. Turshen argues that what working people themselves wanted was radical social and economic change, not environmental engineering or minor social legislation designed to mitigate the worst effects of capital production. The safe disposal of waste and the supply of uninfected water yielded real and measurable reductions in infectious disease, but the inadequacy of the sanitarian approach to health was exposed by the Interdepartmental Committee on Physical Deterioration, which reported in 1904. This committee revealed the enormous extent of ill health associated with poverty and economic exploitation, but rather than resulting in significant changes to the social and economic determinants of health, the committee's findings became the springboard for what is often termed the second, *personal hygiene*, era in public health intervention. Winslow (1952) characterizes this as focusing on education and hygiene, which relocated the responsibility for health improvement with individuals, as opposed to collective community action or state intervention. Newsholme's report of 1913 typifies the then prevailing medical public health attitude that poverty was not in itself a cause of infant deaths (Newsholme, 1936:179–82). Instead, this report maintained that it was the removable evils of 'motherhood ignorance' about infant care and 'poor personal hygiene' that were to blame.

The second stage of public health, occupying the first half of the twentieth century, generated a vast array of clinics and other institutional services to deal with the needs of such vulnerable groups as mothers, infants, school children, and those suffering from particular diseases such as tuberculosis. Inevitably, these services required the employment of a large workforce, with the result that this period became the heyday of the MOH and public health departments of local government. These services brought about greater contact with individuals and families, and 'health education' figured prominently in this work. Increasingly, in the UK the conceptualization of health promotion was dominated by health education in schools. While this state-sponsored health education was underpinned by what we would now call a 'victim blaming' philosophy, an alternative 'liberation and empowerment approach' to health education was also being developed by lobbying groups such as the Children's Minimum Council, the Committee Against Malnutrition and the National Unemployed Workers Movement (Lewis, 1991).

The achievements of public health in the first part of the twentieth century were heavily publicized, not least by figures such as Sir Arthur Newsholme and Sir George Newman, Chief Medical Officers of the time. Both conducted their apologetics in the language of missionary zeal and in a paternalistic spirit, which invited uncritical admiration rather than objective understanding (Newsholme, 1936; Newman, 1939). As in the sanitarian phase, the personal hygiene era brought genuine health gains, but also disadvantages. On the eve of the Second World War, we might characterize public health professionals as bureaucratic, complacent, eugenic and preoccupied with national economic objectives. Worse, in the light of evidence relating to health during the inter-war depression, was not only that public health professionals had made little impact on the problems identified by the Interdepartmental Committee on Physical Deterioration, but also that its elite had manipulated the official statistics to disguise the limitations of its competence (Webster, 1982).

In sum, although the public health establishment during its second phase made every effort to show that its health education services embodied a genuine attempt to empower and liberate the population, this was only true to the most limited extent, and the limitations were recognized by social activists on both the right and left. In the late 1930s new thinking about public health emerged from such sources as the maverick Peckham Health Centre, from the eugenicist Richard Titmuss, and in the form of 'Social Medicine' as advocated by John Ryle (1948). The idea of Social Medicine was to apply a biomedical paradigm to populations. At least in the UK, this was largely an academic construct limited to an intellectual elite and not extending its influence beyond a few university public health departments, with the result that it was ignored by the dominant medical public health establishment.

For a short time planners looked to Social Medicine as the means to revitalize public health. In fact, Social Medicine failed to consolidate its influence, with the result that in the UK epidemiology was its only long-term legacy. This approach is, in turn, being increasingly challenged as embodying a simplistic, biomedical and professionally dominated idea of health (Petersen and Lupton, 1996). Nonetheless, the abortive Social Medicine movement underlined the limitations of the previous era and, in this respect, prepared the ground for health promotion and was one of the factors causing the medical profession to invent the 'new public health'.

Social Medicine accepted that 'health' implied a 'positive' condition, representing much more than freedom from communicable diseases. Achievement of positive health implied a changed attitude to the causes of ill health, involving reference to the 'whole economic, nutritional, occupational, educational, and psychological opportunity or experience of the individual or community' (Ryle, 1948:11–12). The success of Social Medicine depended on a new form of collaboration, in which all medical personnel, 'ordinary health workers and the general public', engaged in genuine teamwork (Leff, 1953: 15). Where necessary, this form of medical intervention also required commitment to social and political action (Crewe, 1945). Although Social Medicine was a British product, it was influenced by thinking elsewhere, particularly in America, and especially by Henry Sigerist, who is generally credited with having been the first to attach special importance to 'health promotion' and to the principles later embodied in the Ottawa Charter (WHO, 1986). Sigerist believed that the primary task of medicine was to 'promote health', and declared that medicine should be seen as a social science. It was 'merely one link in a chain of social welfare institutions', central to which was 'socialised medicine', for which he was also a leading advocate (Sigerist, 1941; Sigerist 1943: 241). Although Social Medicine made little impact in the UK, it was more influential in North America and WHO circles, which ultimately became the main sources for igniting the health promotion movement in the 1970s.

The introduction of the National Health Service in 1948 revolutionized health care in the UK. However, the benefits were distributed unevenly and the activities most relevant to health promotion were located in the most neglected corners of the new service. As one of its most radical changes, the NHS reduced the functions of public health departments, thereby turning the once powerful MOH into a minor functionary in charge of only a small rump of preventive services. While health care was transformed, public health professionals were launched into a phase of disorientation. In a move which seemed symbolic of this collapse of influence, the government abandoned its health centre programme. This had been the only important new function promised to the MOH, and many of the hopes for the realization of Social Medicine's potential had depended upon the creation of health centres (Lewis, 1986; Webster, 1988: 381–8).

At the time of the NHS reorganization of 1974, which completely eliminated local government involvement in the health service, an attempt was made to rescue public health activity from extinction by repackaging it as community medicine, but this too was a failure (Lewis, 1986). In particular, the 1974 changes deprived community medicine specialists of their control of environmental health departments and shifted them back into hospital administration, and also abandoned the annual reports that were a key component of the watchdog role of the MOH. Continuing erosion of confidence led to a further rescue effort in 1988, based on the recommendations of the Acheson Report, which reintroduced public health medicine as the name of the specialty.

Alongside the decline in medically dominated conceptions of public health during the 1960s and 1970s, the empowerment conception of health education continued to grow in influence. It was not until 1976–77 that the UK government issued its first prevention policy documents, but these timid efforts made no permanent mark (Webster, 1996: 660–86). They simply restated the contention that ill health was largely the responsibility of individuals whom, through ignorance, were not looking after themselves. It was implied that ill health, rather than being related to poverty, was attributable to affluent lifestyles. Reflecting the barrenness of thinking about promotion, the commentary on health education of the Royal Commission on the NHS was also entirely lacking in insight (Royal Commission on the NHS, 1979: 44–7). With respect to prevention and promotion, perhaps the most important changes were incidental features of the 1974 NHS reorganization, which gave environmental health officers new professional autonomy under local government, and also established health education as an embryonic specialism in the NHS.

Under the NHS public health medicine limped along with its traditional routines, but it failed to respond to new challenges and it avoided confronting the continuing problems of ill health associated with poverty. The mounting economic crisis of the 1970s prompted new concern about poverty and public health, and stimulated yet another rebirth of Social Medicine. The new social awakening centred around the problem of 'inequality' (Townsend and Bosanquet, 1972). In the field of health, this concern reached its classic expression in the Black Report of 1980 (Townsend and Davidson, 1982). The findings of the Black Report drew together a great deal of evidence that highlighted appalling inequalities in health, maldistribution of resources, and irrational disparities in the provision of seemingly every type of service, including those relating to prevention and promotion (Hart, 1971; Culyer, 1976; Dowling, 1983).

In light of the above brief history, it is not surprising that the impetus for new thinking about public health and health promotion came from outside the UK. The context of this reappraisal was provided by a confluence of forces: first, the rising tide of radical critiques of the medical establishment and the health industry in the western economies; second, a mood of self-criticism within health services concerning their shortcomings, especially with respect to the needs of the poor and the developing world; third, growing concern in western governments over the escalating cost of health care; and finally, the dramatic impact of the oil price rises introduced by OPEC states at the end of 1973. This date marked the end of the golden age of the welfare state, introduced an era of retrenchment, and provoked a rethinking of every aspect of health care. One of the early products of this rethinking was the development of empowerment models of health education and the concept of 'health promotion'.

The three seminal documents that launched the health promotion movement were the Lalonde Report *A New Perspective on the Health of Canadians* (1974), and WHO's *Global Strategy for Health for All by the Year 2000* (1981) and its *Ottawa Charter for Health Promotion* (1986). Together, they set out a vision for health improvement that went beyond sanitation engineering, lifestyle health education and preventive and caring health services, and mark the advent of the *health promotion* phase of public health. Health promotion was concerned principally with empowering citizens so that they could take control of their health and in doing so attain the best possible chance of a full and enjoyable life. The principal methodologies included community development, empowerment, social marketing, advocacy, organizational development and the formulation of integrated health strategies. Bunton (1992) contended that health promotion represented a new form and conception of health intervention. It 'deliberately tried to address issues of power, political, economic and social structures and processes'. MacDonald (1997) suggested that because health promotion is intrinsically revolutionary, governments have, since its conceptualization, been trying by elaborate means to accommodate it and have displayed great ingenuity in appearing to absorb its radical ideas without in reality disrupting the status quo. As governments seek to embed health promotion within the existing medical and health care-dominated agenda, attention is drawn away from the challenges that it presents for society – most radically to set health, rather than the creation of wealth, as the overarching goal of society. As we have seen, this is not a new idea but rather a re-emergence of much earlier calls for health to take priority over wealth creation.

Kelly and Charlton (1995) have, however, pointed out that health promotion is characterized by a difficulty which arises from the failure by its advocates to address their unspoken assumptions about the relationship between social autonomy and social structure. They suggest that this is especially problematic when considering the effects of social inequality on oppressed groups:

> Here the emphasis is on social determinism among the oppressed while maintaining a place for the idea of free will among non-oppressed groups. Empirically this may seem to be the way the world operates, and politically it may make sense to construct things in this way, but theoretically and epistemologically it does not work. (ibid.: 89)

Stevenson and Burke (1991) are even more critical of health promotion, arguing that it weakens struggles for social equity and political change to the extent that 'with its emphasis on organic harmony and consensus among diverse identities and its tendency to develop methodological "resolutions" to political problems, health promotion mystifies rather than clarifies the nature of social barriers to meaningful change' (ibid.: 281).

Health promotion and the 'New Public Health' possess common characteristics. Both are closely associated with the WHO (1981) strategy, and both seem to consist of multiple and disparate strands. Draper believes that the new public health takes a 'comprehensive view of health hazards in the human environment, from the physical, chemical and biological to the socio-economic' (1991: 10). Baum (1990) has argued that the 'new' public health carries the same flaws as many understandings of health promotion, in that it is underpinned by the assumption that change can be achieved through consensus building, while history teaches us that it is conflict and challenges to existing power structures that promote health.

If health promotion and the new public health have a major distinguishing feature, it would appear to be the conviction that health is a right – as opposed to older ideas of health as a necessity for national efficiency, or as a moral duty of citizens. However, even this claim does not withstand critical examination. The 'health as a right' concept can be traced back for thousands of years and, like 'health as a means to efficient production', represents a recurrent theme. The health as a right concept has, however, continuously been subordinated to a more politically and capital-sensitive paradigm which emphasizes individual and environment solutions to poor health over social and economic ones.

Yet it is possible to make an even more critical assessment of the new public health movement. It is arguable that the new public health – a concept developed largely by medical practitioners working in the public health field – represents an assault by the medical profession, intent on recapturing the commanding heights which were lost to the globally developed and more inclusive notion of health promotion. Evidence of this reassertion of public health is evident in much of the UK government's recent health strategy. The term health promotion is noticeable by its absence, despite the fact that internationally the phrase is used as an umbrella term that includes the subset of public health. As indicated in the quotation from Alan Milburn above, it seems that the case for interdisciplinary and intersectoral partnerships to promote health is now accepted by the UK government. The recently established Health Development Agency in England seems to be a concrete expression of this acceptance, although only time will tell whether the agency will receive the governmental support it needs to be effective.

The public health and health promotion professions embody – and tolerate – conflicting ideas of why and how health should and could be improved. The meaning of public health and health promotion are themselves contested and open to a range of understandings. The origins of these conflicts lie in the contested nature of health itself, of the causes of ill health, of the methods for reducing ill health and promoting well-being, and fundamentally, in the motivation for such interventions. The historical record suggests that one expression of these conflicts has been through the cyclical invention, abandonment and reinvention of the 'social model' of health and disease which, when advocated, quickly falls out of favour due to the fact that it inevitably brings its supporters into direct conflict with the state and existing economic interests. Alongside this, the history of public health has also been one of a long battle for occupational domination by the medical profession. Given a widespread acceptance of the complexity of improving health, and the UK government's moves to develop multidisciplinary public health leadership, the traditional hegemony of the medical profession is clearly no longer sustainable.

The promotion of health depends upon the engagement of a wide number of sectors and professions. Public health promotion has always been, and remains, a collective activity. Only if we are prepared to recognize the historic conflict, and the contested nature of health promotion and public health, will it be possible to develop a deeper understanding of how the battle could be more effectively fought on behalf of those currently deprived of their rights to health. In the light of history, it is clear that the fundamental test of health promotion is yet to come as it struggles to exercise any influence at all in a world increasingly shaped by global economic forces.

1.1

PRACTISING HEALTH FOR ALL IN THE UK

Maddy Halliday

This chapter outlines the key strengths and weaknesses of the Health For All (HFA) strategy and the challenges faced by those trying to work within it in the UK. The chapter discusses two short case studies.

HEALTH FOR ALL AND HEALTH 21

HFA is the World Health Organisation's global public health strategy, with different versions serving different world regions such as Europe, the Americas and Africa. The HFA regional strategy for Europe is the one which relates to the UK. The original HFA strategy was developed in the late 1970s (WHO, 1981, 1985), but during the 1990s was updated and further developed to become Health 21, a new strategy for the 21st century (WHO, 1999a). Health 21 represents a challenging approach to health, informed by debates within diverse health and social movements across the world (see Box 1.1.1).

BOX 1.1.1 HEALTH 21: A CHALLENGING STRATEGY FOR HEALTH IN THE TWENTY-FIRST CENTURY

Visionary – presenting desirable goals for improving health, embracing physical, mental and social well-being, within a social–ecological approach to public health
Value-based – expressing a commitment to social justice, equity, participation and other progressive 'liberal' values
Evidence-based – informed by an understanding of the holistic and complex nature of health, its biological, social and environmental determinants and the range of political, social and technical interventions necessary to protect and promote health
Practical – offering a coherent framework for the development of international, national and local health policies, programmes and services

Over the past 20 years HFA has inspired a world-wide movement, expressed most strongly through primary health care initiatives in developing nations and WHO's Healthy Cities Projects, which have been established across Europe and globally.

Health 21 builds on this and provides stronger links to the United Nations' other 'big' strategy – Agenda 21, the global and local strategy for sustainable development (United Nations, 1992b). Health 21, as its predecessor, is formally endorsed by member states of the UN, including the UK.

While there are many positive aspects to HFA/Health 21, there are also weaknesses in the strategy and, despite its huge support, its success is debatable given that health indicators in many parts of the world, particularly Africa and Eastern Europe, have deteriorated rather than improved over the past 20 years. The problem for HFA is that the main social, economic and environmental determinants of health are heavily influenced by the structures and organizations of global capitalism, which take little notice of human health or ecological consequences. As do all visionary, desirable expressions of human intent, such as the Declaration of Human Rights and Agenda 21, HFA needs the support of political and civil society, and particularly of those who hold the most power. Without such support, strategies such as HFA remain simply statements of desires. Given that WHO is a relatively weak UN agency, it has not been able to influence strongly the policies and practice of powerful international agencies, multinationals and nation–states.

HFA has inspired the support of many national and local groups and professionals, but it has barely influenced mainstream socio-economic policy. Powerful international agencies such as the International Monetary Fund and the World Trade Organisation pursue policies which generally increase wealth for a few while increasing poverty and environmental degradation for many, particularly people in developing nations. Some nation–states, including the UK, have also pursued social and economic policies which have increased health inequality (Department of Health, 1999a; Mitchell et al., 2000). Other nations have been involved in protracted wars, reversing many decades of health improvement.

Does this mean that HFA/Health 21 has failed? I would say it has not. It could be accused of being naïve in its presentation, in that it does not explicitly articulate the political reality of improving health, but of course if it did so, nation–states and international agencies would not sign up to it. HFA is a balancing act. It presents a visionary way forward in a way which secures formal support from powerful nations and bodies and which also encourages a global 'grass-roots' movement to emerge, working to achieve its goals (WHO, 1998). In this way HFA might gradually, over decades, achieve a deep-rooted change in attitudes, policy and practice. The key question is, given the threat to human health of global warming, whether we have time left to achieve such change. In the light of available evidence, it is uncertain whether we do. Rather than blame HFA for its failure, the real problem is the human-created system – capitalism – that is destroying the life support systems on which we depend.

HEALTH FOR ALL IN THE UK

Over the past 20 years in the UK there has been only moderate engagement with HFA by government, health agencies and other bodies. There are a number reasons for this relative neglect. First, HFA represents a paradigm shift in terms of its approach to health. Health 21 is consistent with the 'new public health' but not mainstream approaches to health, which are still dominated by a bio-medical approach. Second, the political values of successive Conservative governments between 1979–97 were explicitly opposed to the liberal values of HFA. Third, there has generally been low awareness and understanding of HFA within the statutory, professional, academic and voluntary sectors as, given the above factors, it has not attracted sufficient support and resources to enable effective promotion, dissemination and implementation. And finally, unlike Agenda 21, HFA has received little media interest in the UK (Halliday, 1994).

Despite these difficulties, grass-roots support for HFA in the UK grew during the 1980s and 1990s, particularly among 'progressive' health practitioners and community groups, often leading to the formation of Healthy City and Health For All projects. In 1988 the UK Health For All Network (UKHFAN) was formed as a membership organization for HFA/Healthy City projects. Despite considerable funding difficulties, the UKHFAN has continued to provide a range of services and activities. In 1987 the UK Public Health Association was formed, and while the UKPHA is not an explicit HFA organization, its philosophy and approach to public health are informed by HFA and many PHA members are actively involved in local HFA initiatives.

The public health policy of the New Labour government (Department of Health, 1999b; Secretary of State for Scotland, 1999) reflects some understanding and support for HFA and the new public health, although it does not adequately apply its approach and strengths. This policy shift can be attributed, at least in part, to the strength of the growing new public health movement in the UK as represented by the UKPHA and UKHFAN, although the government does not readily acknowledge this. Nonetheless, the change of government has provided, for the first time in 20 years, a real chance to build support for Health 21 in the UK.

The national picture outlined above is also found at local level in the UK, where a large number of HFA/Healthy City initiatives have struggled to influence health policy and practice and improve health. The two case studies which follow illustrate this experience.

GLASGOW HEALTHY CITY PARTNERSHIP: LESSONS FOR THE PUBLIC HEALTH MOVEMENT

Glasgow Healthy City Partnership was established in 1996, building on its predecessor Glasgow Healthy City Project. From 1988 onwards, both the project and the successor partnership had a WHO Healthy City designation.

The Partnership serves the population of Glasgow, which is now around 660,000. Glasgow's population has some of the best and worst health in Scotland and the UK, reflecting patterns of wealth and deprivation in the city. Poor health is particularly marked in Glasgow, as ten of its electoral wards have the highest premature mortality rate in the UK. Not surprisingly, these wards also experience severe social and economic deprivation on a wide range of indicators including unemployment, receipt of benefits and free school meals, single parent families, and post-16 education (Sherwood and Halliday, 1998).

Poverty and poor health in Glasgow are not new, nor is its position as bottom of the UK's health league table. These problems go back to the development of Glasgow as a major industrial city 150 years ago, which brought low wages, pollution and unsanitary conditions. While living conditions and pollution improved dramatically during the twentieth century, Glasgow's economic fortunes ebbed and flowed with periods of high and low unemployment. The progressive collapse of Glasgow's main industries from the 1970s (shipbuilding and textiles) led to major social and economic problems, reflected in its poor health profile.

In the past 25 years the city council and economic development agencies have tried to improve Glasgow's economic fortunes, with some success. Glasgow now is the second biggest shopping centre in the UK outside London and is a major site for service industries. Despite this, many of the new jobs have been taken by people living in more affluent areas outside Glasgow, while unemployment and associated social problems in the deprived communities remain prevalent. Regeneration initiatives in Glasgow continue to try to solve these problems, with partial success.

The result of this situation is continued poor health and this is the challenge which led to the Glasgow Healthy City Project and then the partnership. After 12 years the project/partnership could be credited with some successes. It has raised awareness of the health problems which Glasgow faces, and it has improved understanding of the determinants of health and the measures necessary to improve health. It has supported joint working between public and voluntary agencies, the development of community health projects across the city and, more recently development of proposals for Healthy Living Centres. It has also secured the integration of health goals within the city regeneration strategies and programmes, and has developed a range of linked health programmes, including women's health, tobacco and child health.

But it has achieved much less than would have been possible without a multitude of obstacles, similar to those experienced by HFA at international and national level and other HFA/Healthy City projects in the UK. First, given the huge health challenge in Glasgow, the project/partnership were not established with sufficient authority, power or resources. This is illustrated by the relatively low grading for the initiative's co-ordinator, its small staff team and modest development budget. Over the years, the success of the initiative enabled its resource base to be protected during times of cuts and even led to some increase in resources, but progress was slowed by the poor resource base relative to the task. Second, while it was easy to secure formal support from Glasgow's health board and the city council, this did not lead to meaningful support and engagement by these organizations as a whole. Project/partnership staff and allies had to spend many years 'working the system' to build support, but this could quickly be undone with political and key staff changes. With notable exceptions, most politicians and senior management in both organizations failed to promote or support the initiative in a proactive manner. Third, until the election of the 1997 New Labour government, the initiative had to work to improve health locally in a hostile national environment. This made it very difficult to achieve anything but marginal gains.

From the author's experience and various research and evaluation initiatives, these three issues – lack of power and resources; organizational failure to engage; hostile national policy environment – reflect the main obstacles to successful local HFA/Healthy City initiatives in the UK. Although the national policy environment has improved to some extent (Hamer and Ross, 2000), issues of power, resources and organizational failure remain. These problems affect not only HFA/Healthy City initiatives, but also the Health Action Zones in England. The reason for these problems is complex but there are three important contributors: the dominance of a bio-medical approach to health generally makes it hard for alternative perspectives on health to secure support and resources; correspondingly, the dominance of the NHS in health planning and the relatively weak role of local government make it difficult to develop an inter-agency public health strategy; and the poor understanding of public health issues both in and outside the NHS leads to a lack of motivation to engage with HFA/Healthy Cities.

There are a number of measures which could improve matters. Access to public health learning opportunities should be improved, both in mainstream education and occupationally-based training schemes, with development of a multi-disciplinary approach to public health covering a range of professions. Such an approach should include a range of professional groups within the NHS, local government, voluntary sector and academia. The UK Multi-disciplinary Public Health Forum is arguing for such developments, although is still fairly focused on the NHS. Formal joint responsibility for public health planning between the NHS and local government is needed, with better integration of health dimensions into public policy and plans, such as community planning. More broadly, we need improved public education about the creation of health and its links to sustainable development, to increase awareness and influence political debate and action.

A few organizations in the UK, such as the UK Public Health Association, the Society for Health Promotion Specialists and the UK Health For All Network, are arguing for such change. They are supported, to varying degrees, by public sector, union and professional organizations such as the Faculty for Public Health, Institution of Environmental Health Officers and local government associations. Sadly, however, it is unlikely that Health For All in the UK will ever be able to realize its potential without broader public and political support. I hope, in time, organizations such as those cited above are able to help foster the public interest and political will for such changes to be realized.

HEALTHY SHEFFIELD[1]

Sheffield is a city of almost half a million people, well known for its industrial pre-eminence in the nineteenth and early twentieth centuries. Since the 1970s economic decline has led to widening inequalities within the city, closely related to the geographic divisions of the city. The east of Sheffield contains many of the large public sector housing estates that provided the labour force for the steel industry. Intermingled with these are smaller areas of private sector housing which are home to many of the economic migrants recruited to the city in the boom years from Pakistan, the Yemen and the Caribbean. On the west of Sheffield most of the middle class live: academics, public sector managers, and those who manage and own the more successful private sector businesses. Since the 1970s the city has under-performed in economic, educational and health terms but while the west of the city compares well to successful areas elsewhere, the east side has some of the poorest wards nationally.

The strategy of city leaders has emphasized economic regeneration. This approach, which has been championed by the city's strategic partnership 'Sheffield First', can be summarized as building on existing specialist expertise, attracting new businesses and ensuring that the city has an educated and skilled workforce. Although some elements of the strategy focus on inequality, this is within the context of economic regeneration.

THE HEALTH FOR ALL APPROACH IN SHEFFIELD

Sheffield has had a Health For All project since 1987, jointly funded over the years by a range of partners including the health sector, local government, and the academic and voluntary sector. Since it began there have been six co-ordinators, which perhaps indicates the stresses and frustrations associated with the work. For much of its existence, the Healthy Sheffield partnership existed outside of mainstream activity – one local director of public health described it as a 'guerrilla organization'. Whether its aims and methods were ever as radical as this implies is questionable, but it certainly provided an alternative analysis that:

- promoted a multi-sectoral approach to tackling inequalities;
- developed techniques for involving the socially excluded in decision-making;
- piloted local community development interventions;
- suggested a different set of priorities to those promoted by the establishment at a local and national level.

Recently Healthy Sheffield has changed again. It was commissioned to work with the director of public health to redesign the city's health partnership, seeking to bring together the strategic planning of health services with policies addressing the root causes of ill health. This approach has seen Healthy Sheffield being subsumed within a broader health partnership – 'Sheffield First for Health'. The advantages and disadvantages of this are that advocates of Health for All principles are at the table but their voice remains weak. In the context of national and local concerns the priority remains the performance of the health and social care sectors. In its current manifestation the healthy city office – costing £100,000 annually compared to the £500m spent by the health sector in Sheffield – continues to provide services that remain consistent with Health For

All principles. The approach taken by the Healthy City team consists of the following elements:

- *Partnership* – supporting the development of effective partnership working at a strategic level, with an emphasis on ensuring the active engagement of the voluntary and community sectors.
- *Resources* – providing the resources for effective partnership working, these include ensuring that demographic information is presented in a manner that identifies links between exclusion and ill health and producing up-to-date information on multi-sectoral activity.
- *Models* – developing and promoting models that provide alternatives to purely medical interventions, in particular, ones that break down cultural and professional barriers between the socially excluded and professional service providers.
- *Strategies* – developing strategies to address the root causes of ill health by bringing together policy-makers (particularly those responsible for addressing social exclusion) to develop a joined-up approach that targets excluded communities. An important element of this work is developing health impact assessment methodology not just as a tool to evaluate major policy change but also as a mechanism to give the non-health sector confidence in the contribution that it can make.

In summary, we are concerned with working at the interface of organizations and interest groups. By providing and developing these tools the team seeks to support statutory agencies, addressing their concern to engage staff and community members in their work, at the same time as keeping the door open for community members to represent their interests and put pressure on services.

NOTE

1 This case study was written by Mark Gamsu.

1.2

BUILDING A UK PUBLIC HEALTH MOVEMENT: A PHOENIX FROM THE ASHES?

Geof Rayner

From campaigns to alleviate third world debt to the protection of rare species, citizens' movements have come alive in the UK – and across the world – in the past 20 years. But one movement – the public health movement – has been slower to ignite, despite many urgent reasons for it to do so. How might a mass movement be rekindled? Is there anything to learn from the environmental movement and consumer movement?

Environmental and consumer campaigning 'took off' in the last quarter of the twentieth century. The first was driven by a public perception that neither states nor international institutions were doing enough to protect the planet from unbridled industrialization and urbanization. In fact, many concluded, international institutions like the World Trade Organisation were part of the problem. The harmful results were everywhere: they encompassed the local – a rural landscape consumed by housing, town bypass roads, fears of contaminated foods – and the global – the devastation of natural habitats with early signs of imbalance and exhaustion to the earth's fragile ecosystem. Environmentalism became a common cause for those at either end of the political spectrum.

All of this was generated by a growing perception that environmental threats touched everyone. But movements are also born of activists, not of passive members. Opinion studies suggested that around one in five adults (18 per cent) could be described as 'environmental activists' (defined as people who have carried out five or more 'green' behaviours in the previous two years) while a slightly larger proportion (24 per cent) avoided using the services or products of companies that they felt had a poor environmental record (MORI, 1996). Of course, a much wider section of society blended 'a degree' of environmentalism with 'a degree' of consumerism, and the question of the core values of the consumer movement was uncertain. While the *avante garde* of consumers may have seen themselves as environmentalists, mainstream consumers merely sought out 'good value'. Although the income gap between top and bottom earners had grown ever greater, the comfortable middle had grown too, with profound implications not only for political parties but for social movements.

Such movements encompassed many different motivations in their membership and were vehicles for, or connected to, a wide span of personal beliefs. Whatever the combination of elements in play, the appeal was strong enough to attract subscriptions on a mass scale. Friends of the Earth, Greenpeace, the Royal Society for the Protection of Birds, to name but three, attracted over a million members between them. The consumer movement was different. Perhaps recognizing that consumers as a whole lacked an altruistic vision, the Consumers' Association sought to offer more concrete benefits, such as comparative reviews of goods and services, and even holidays. Surprisingly, perhaps, this instinct to offer value for money – even to the extent of organizing lower car prices (with obvious environmental implications) provided few limits to the association's broader policy advocacy.

Alongside these high points of citizen activism, where exactly did the public health movement stand? In Victorian times, it seemed fairly clear: public health was tightly joined to both environmentalism and consumerism, forming part of an array of social forces encompassing citizens' groups, rising professions, progressive local authorities, town planners, sanitarians, co-operators, temperance advocates, lobbyists for clean food, and many others. By the last quarter of the twentieth century, however, public health had lost any appeal it may have had. The pejorative term 'nanny state' conjured up an image of spoon-fed do-gooding at a time when, according to opponents, rugged individualism was required. Compare this with the vitality of some elements of environmentalism, with their publicity-conscious tree climbing, tunnel digging and polluter teasing.

Anyone surveying the UK for mass-scale, vision-driven campaigning focusing on public health and well-being would have been disappointed. Although, in the 1990s, there were organizations that wanted to develop a profile like that of Friends of the Earth or Greenpeace – for example, the Public Health Alliance, the Association for Public Health or UK Health For All Network – they lacked both resources and impact. This is not to say that health campaigning was invisible. On the contrary, messages about cancer, heart disease, HIV/AIDS, drugs, safe driving, and so on were prevalent. Professional and voluntary health-related organizations abounded. So why hadn't a movement developed? The failure of the public health movement to offer much more than the sum of its parts requires some explanation and, in fact, there are several.

One reason is historic, originating in the way public health campaigners had worked from their earliest days. Voluntary associations dedicated to eradicating a specific disease or tackling a particular health threat have been a core part of the public health movement in the UK and abroad since its earliest days (Teller, 1988). Part of the success of public health action has been the result of the diverse disciplines it incorporated, including epidemiological, ecological, engineering, sanitary, and lifestyle perspectives. Public health activism has long had a scientific and modernizing flavour, and the association with scientific medicine, statistical measurement and research was an important means for establishing its case in the political arena, but in truth early public health measures were built as much on inspiration as on science.

But there may also have been a negative side to the 'single issue' approach. Over time, campaigners competing for public support sought to differentiate themselves from one another with the result that, in public debate, a holistic understanding of health was undermined. What caused the illness which 'heart' campaigns, for example, were addressing? Was it smoking, fatty food, lack of exercise, or was the real problem lack of diagnostic facilities or acute care beds? The public could be forgiven for being confused.

'Nannyism' may also have been a factor in explaining the movement's poor appeal. Since its earliest days, public health thinking had embraced the regulatory state, beginning with the sanitary revolution, which had embedded public health institutionally and professionally within the central and local state. There was also, to put it crudely, a 'health police' function, particularly in the early years of sexually transmitted disease prevention. To many people – especially the poor – many public health practices had an undesirable supervisory strand: less facilitation of better health or campaigning about injustices, more attempted control of lifestyle. In our modern, less deferential era, such approaches have become unsustainable.

A third reason was the urge among public health campaigners for respectability and professionalism. When they started, many of the professional bodies and multidisciplinary associations had a radical edge, but over time a narrowing of vision and role led to a conservative focus on ensuring benefits to members, such as professional accreditation, career-building or education.

If the public health movement had lost the plot, had anyone noticed? By the end of the Second World War public health measures were taken for granted, established in statute and practice. Professional groups jostled for influence and, occasionally, lifted their heads above the parapet to utter polite words of protest. In some cases, associations made eloquent attempts to restate their vision (Chartered Institute of Environmental Health, 1999). The resurgence of a movement was encouraged by the emergence of several issues which were being actively ignored by government: extensive health inequalities, repeated concerns over food quality, the growing power of anti-health forces, led by the tobacco industry, and evidence of a gradual decline in social and community infrastructure.

At the same time, questions were being raised about the ability of health services to cure every ill. The health improvements which had been the success stories of the past century were slowing, and some were even reversing. For example, in Wales 14 per cent of 15-year-old boys and 22 per cent of 15-year-old girls smoked at least weekly in 1989–90; by 1993–94 the figures had risen to 18 per cent and 27 per cent, respectively. In addition, income inequality widened dramatically: in 1979–80 the proportion of households receiving below 40 per cent of mean average income was under 5 per cent. By 1996–97, it was almost 15 per cent. The UK was becoming a service and information-based economy, in which highly paid jobs contrasted with low-paid, non-routine jobs undertaken by women, school leavers, students and older, pre-retired men – the latter a group whose health has improved least over the past 40 years. Poverty in the UK, amidst mass affluence, cannot be ignored.

Through all the social, economic and cultural changes single issue campaigns persisted, and some even thrived. Food became the most prominent focus for public health campaigning in the UK. Evidence emerged not only that families were losing skills in cooking and nutrition but that our industrially driven food industry was encouraging obesity. However, most public attention was focused on food scares. Bovine Spongiform Encephalopathy (BSE) was first identified as a disease of cattle in 1986 and it was not until a decade later that it was linked to new variant Creutzfeldt-Jakob Disease (nvCJD), prompting a £4 billion 'rescue' involving the mass slaughter of herds. The later official BSE inquiry confirmed the lassitude of official thought and action, with civil servants in MAFF presenting a continually optimistic view of the evidence, and the inability of Department of Health officials to enforce public health priorities (Phillips, 2000).

Not only was public confidence in British meat found wanting, but also, progressively, confidence in government science. As a direct consequence of BSE and later concerns over genetically modified organisms, opinion polls have demonstrated that scientists in voluntary campaigns were held in higher esteem than official scientists.

A further – and possibly dominant – factor underlying the difficulties facing the public health movement in the post-war period may be the 'medicalization' of health. Although medical science never claimed that it would cure all ills and most doctors would emphasize the importance of living conditions in improving health, medicine has crowded out other models of intervention. During the twentieth century the belief grew that solutions to health problems could be scientifically discovered in the laboratory, prescribed, purchased, or to use the epithet increasingly common to the NHS, 'delivered'.

So far, mostly the obstacles have been considered. What are the opportunities for the growth of the public health movement? There is no public disinterest in health: on the contrary, judged by opinion polls health is consistently a highly rated concern for the population. When MORI asked people to judge which, among a list of ten or so things that might be 'most important for you personally in determining how happy or unhappy you are in general these days', 'health' was rated first (59 per cent), followed by 'family life' (41 per cent), 'marriage/partner' (35 per cent) and 'job/employment' (31 per cent). These came far ahead of education received (7 per cent), housing conditions (9 per cent) or even financial condition/money (25 per cent) (Worcester, 1998).

If these values are widely shared, they might encourage optimism about the rebirth of a public health movement. Unfortunately, however, the beliefs which underlie these responses are contradictory. The influence of medicalization has already been mentioned: when a group of 18 to 24-year-olds were asked to list the greatest achievements of the twentieth century, the lunar landing came third, the defeat of Hitler second and the winner was ... the first heart transplant. Another issue related to health beliefs is that we are ill-acquainted with conceptualizing risk. For example, we disregard the safety of the mundane. We discount serious risks because we face them every day. We accept smoking, although it is the greatest preventable cause of disease, but we worry about the risks of rail travel – many times safer than road transport – because tragic and shocking rail accidents speak to our fears of not being in control (the car, by contrast, is seen almost as an extension of ourselves). Ironically, the corollary is also true: our faith in doctors may be linked to the fact that we do not tend to come into contact with them very often against the observance of a pervasive ethic of security in medicine.

Thus health belief harbours a central paradox: health is interpreted in terms of more apparently abstract threats – things read about in the press, the observable living environment, how we feel, and powerful images of the role of medicine. These do not fit together or match up. The abstract threats are far removed and breed anxiety; medicine can do little about the factors which influence our health and well-being.

Against this background, the principles, beliefs, and approaches of the modern public health movement, as codified in creeds like Health For All, are remote and unfamiliar. Once understood, they still seem difficult for us to make use of individually, because they refer to the workings and structure of society. Even when the idea of healthy public policy has a reference point at an individual level – the benefits of walking as part of a sustainable transport policy, for example – society prepares us with counter-beliefs. While the car is now designed and sold with strong appeal to our fantasies, the alternatives – walking, or reliable trains – appeal only to our needs.

So how can the public health movement move forward? It is clear that the movement carries a lot of heavy baggage from the past; its vision has dimmed and become obscure to the public; it has tendencies to tribal divisions and professional infighting; and it has often been aligned with the regulatory state. Since the environmental and consumer movements have tapped public concerns in ways in which public health has not, are there lessons there which should be learnt? Or are there other changes which might support the rebirth of a public health movement?

Let us deal with the last question first: because the public health movement is more institutional in character it is important to link what it does with what government thinks. The *Health of the Nation* strategy (Department of Health, 1992) was launched by a Conservative government in 1990, and the Labour government's *Saving Lives: Our Healthier Nation* (Department of Health, 1999b) was launched eight years later. Key developments in Labour's approach included the emphasis on tackling inequality (later followed up in Sir Donald Acheson's (1998) *Report of the Independent Inquiry into Inequalities in Health*), the emphasis on communities, better 'joining up' of government actions, and the commitment to multi-disciplinary actions. Although *Saving Lives* rejected the individualistic focus of *Health of the Nation*, glaring defects remained. Local authorities were given scant attention; the role of industry and the press was ignored, while the role of the NHS – and the medical model of health – was over-emphasized. Nevertheless, it was an advance. *Saving Lives* understood that health is influenced by factors that go beyond the biological and individual: social, economic and political influences – the so-called determinants of health – are seen as critically important. Yet it established targets and outlined ways of achieving them that focused exclusively on health trends and potential risks, rather than the social and cultural context within which healthy public policy could be developed.

Because action on health inequalities, the physical and social regeneration of neighbourhoods, and the modernization of professional practice is now central to government across the UK (albeit with national variations), it brings government strictures on public services into reasonable proximity with the arguments of the public health movement. Coincidentally, the launch of *Saving Lives* occurred at almost the same time as the launch of the new combined public health association, the UK Public Health Association (UKPHA). The association's purpose was, in part, to work with the grain of these developments in government thinking, at the same time as attracting a new constituency of workers who saw a public health component to their job, and also to appeal to a wider audience – voluntary campaigners and others – as concerns about health issues grew.

Although the fact that environmentalism and consumerism have attracted so many supporters can encourage this new association and the movement associated with it, its area of work and capacity to bring in members are different. Perhaps, in some respects, it can do its job better. While environmentalists have not fought shy of using scare tactics (phrases such as 'Frankenstein foods', for example), the fact that the public health movement includes many (like nutritionists) who work with people, rather than just issues, gives it a strong reality test. The arguments concern people and communities rather than inanimate nature, so for the 'new' public health movement people, not the environment, come first.

Summing up, the aims of the public health movement must be:

- to develop and spread a vision of a healthier society – and not simply add to 'health scares';
- to promote the view that health is more than about waiting lists, hospitals and visits to the doctor – while not denigrating medicine, encouraging it to see the bigger picture;
- to argue for healthy public policy – across transport, food, employment, etc.;
- to build support for public health thinking among employees of the NHS and local government;
- to engage the voluntary sector, the environmental movement, the consumer movement, the professions and the public;
- to campaign for 'health justice' by showing the full consequences of health inequalities;
- to combat anti-health forces, presenting an alternative, sustainable health perspective not just across the UK but also in Europe and all points beyond.

1.3

PROMOTING SOCIAL AND COMMUNITY DEVELOPMENT IN SHEFFIELD: A REFLECTION OF TEN YEARS' WORK

Lee Adams and Frances Cunning

This chapter reflects on ten years of promoting health in Sheffield, where we managed a health authority department and worked in partnership with a range of agencies, notably Sheffield City Council. We will show how we tried, explicitly, to draw upon, develop and articulate a coherent set of principles and evidence base for our work, and will describe how this work developed.

For much of the ten years in question, from 1989 to 1999, we were working under a Conservative government, but we also experienced a year or so of a New Labour administration, and will show how national policy impacted on our work at local level. Much of our inspiration came from other sources, especially WHO's Health For All (HFA) programme (WHO, 1981), and its local expression in Healthy Sheffield. We were also heavily influenced by our own backgrounds and training, the evidence on inequalities in health and their causes, the views of local people, professionals and our staff, who came from diverse backgrounds, including social science, nursing, teaching, research and medical work. We shared strong values consistent with those of HFA, but developed them further locally. We must also pay a debt of gratitude to other health promotion specialists and community development and health activists who inspired us. We were both active in the Society of Health Promotion and Health Education Specialists and developed a radical perspective which drew on sociology and social policy, political science, ecology and sustainable development, and applied these to health.

THE THEORETICAL AND EVIDENCE BASE

In 1988 we inherited a small department of health promotion with a mixed reputation, unclear role and no connection to the new healthy city initiative, Healthy Sheffield, described in a previous contribution. We were fortunate in having some excellent staff, far-sighted management and the support of the health authority. It was therefore possible to set out a vision, recruit new staff, and redesign our approach. At the same time we began to develop a working relationship with colleagues in Sheffield City Council and the voluntary sector.

At its peak the department had over 40 staff, and the work described below is a testament to their efforts and the collective philosophy we hold.

We would describe the approach which evolved as a social model of health. We believe that many things – primarily social, economic and environmental factors – influence health. We were also motivated by the very obvious inequalities in health across Sheffield. In response to the research evidence available (Marmot and McDowell, 1986; Blane et al. 1990; Wilkinson, 1996) we focused our efforts on the root causes of ill health. Although we accepted the limitations of the Health For All strategy – an essentially reformist approach which we felt could not achieve its goals – its focus on prerequisites for health and the principles of partnership, community participation and equity were still very radical in the late 1980s. It was rare for a health promotion unit (as we were then called) to take this approach (Adams, 1993), which was very much against the mainstream of national policy (Thomas, 1993).

We also looked to the principles of the Ottawa Charter, an influential statement of good practice that emerged from a WHO health promotion conference in 1986 (WHO, 1986). The Ottawa Charter suggested that health promotion work should operate in several distinct domains: changing public policy, creating supportive environments, strengthening community action, developing personal skills, and re-orienting health services. It also set out three ways in which health could be promoted: through advocacy, empowering people to argue for rights and opportunities; enablement, to reduce inequalities; and mediation, working across sectors. This was a touchstone for us in developing our approach, and still has great relevance today.

Over ten years, with our departmental colleagues, we continually discussed our theory base and focus, trying to refine what we did to achieve our aims. By the mid-1990s, based on these discussions, we had reached the following definition:

> The promotion of health is concerned with maximizing individuals' and communities' involvement in improving and protecting their quality of life and well-being. Health promotion aims to address equity in health, the risks to health, sustainable environments conducive to health, and the empowerment of individuals and communities by contributing to healthy public policy, advocating for health, enabling skills development and education.

While none of us were entirely satisfied with this, it does capture some of our thinking at the time. By then we had picked up further influences, including work on tackling poverty and health (Benzeval et al., 1995), a seminar on the development of theory (Adams and Armstrong, 1996) and sustainable development (United Nations, 1992b), all of which reinforced our focus on poverty and renewed our commitment to action, with a more environmental approach to our work.

By 1998, it was possible to set out a model which evolved both from our practice and from what we felt was a strong evidence base. Essentially there were three strands to the model: *levels* of work, *principles* and *domains*. In order to be effective, we believe that work for health needs to be undertaken at different levels. In Sheffield we used five levels, based on the work of Benzeval et al. (1995) and the Ottawa Charter (WHO, 1986), as follows:

- working to influence national and international social, economic and environment policy;
- working to change local policy and environments;
- working to change and improve local services;
- working with communities, taking a community development approach;
- working to promote the health of individuals.

The principles were those we helped to develop at Penrith (Adams and Armstrong, 1996):

- the right for individuals to live in a society where health is promoted and protected;
- equity, concerned with the redistribution of power and resources, to enable the reduction/elimination of inequalities;
- empowering or enabling people to have control over their lives and health: community development helps in this process; we acknowledge some people needed practical help, support and advocacy for this to be achieved;
- anti-oppressive, challenging systems, services, policies and people who oppress and discriminate against others on grounds of race, class, ethnicity, sexuality, gender, ability or age;
- inclusive and democratic, involving people as much as possible in determining needs, planning and action;
- focused on well-being and development, not illness or parts of the body: a holistic approach based upon felt needs, avoiding blaming individuals for ill health over which they have no control;
- futurity: regard for the health of those not yet born;
- acknowledgement of the limits of what can be achieved at local level: action must take place at national and increasingly international levels.
- spirituality, the process of individuals and groups developing their own sense of place in the world, how they connect with all life and across generations, and with the non-material.

The domains we considered to be the 'building blocks' for health included housing, warmth, positive relationships, education, freedom from violence, good food, meaningful and safe work, a healthy environment, support, sense of purpose and self-esteem. Similar aspirations can be found in the manifestos of various organizations, such as Oxfam, and the UK Public Health Association, suggesting a consensus on basic health rights.

These three strands influenced our work and, as two staff wrote in 1994, the action flowing from these was to 'build up the building blocks for health, empower individually and collectively for people to get the most out of the systems and services, empower collectively to challenge the structures that determined their health experience'(Adams and Pintus, 1994).

THE POLICY CONTEXT

It is interesting – even amazing – that we were able to undertake this work, with the approach outlined above underpinning it explicitly, given such a hostile political and professional climate. Perhaps Sheffield's radical history, the chartist and anarchist movements of past centuries and a radical local government, including health campaigns in the 1980s, enabled us to argue for a social approach to health. Certainly, we and many of the people we worked with had been attracted to Sheffield because of this reputation.

The national context of the NHS influenced us in several ways. The creation of the internal market in the NHS in 1991 and the first national public health strategy *Health of the Nation* (Department of Health, 1992) both had a major impact. To ensure that we maintained a strategic focus we became very involved in commissioning both health services and health promotion work from hospitals, community health services and the voluntary sector, rather than leave the health authority and become 'service providers' ourselves.

The *Health of the Nation* was a huge step forward in legitimizing public health activity but its focus on individual lifestyle and neglect of a social understanding of health were disappointing. This did not support our approach, so that our work had to encompass issues such as skin cancer prevention and other disease-based activity, which we tried to tackle in the ways described above. We also tried to ensure that local health services also did so, for example, our contracts all required anti-poverty work. However, broad holistic approaches to women's health, for example, had to be refocused on parts of women's bodies with the potential for disease. But we still managed to progress holistic work such as a maternal health strategy that emphasized prevention, partnership, and a woman-centred approach as well as service provision. Other Conservative government initiatives such as *Local Voices* (NHS Management Executive, 1992) – increasing patient and community involvement – and moves towards a 'primary care-led NHS' provided some opportunities for radical practice. For example, we initiated a comprehensive health authority strategy for community participation, and helped draw up a community development strategy with one primary care commissioning group. It was a case of working to fulfil government demand, but in such a way as to remain true to our principles.

In 1997, with a change of government, we had high hopes for public health becoming a national priority. The way ahead was set out in the White Paper *The New NHS – Modern, Dependable* (Department of Health, 1997) and later in the public health strategy *Saving Lives: Our Healthier Nation* (Department of Health, 1999b). The commitment to reducing inequalities, and indeed eliminating child poverty in 20 years, was welcome and the proposal for primary care groups and trusts to have responsibilities in public health as well as health care was encouraging. In addition, new powers for local authorities to promote social, economic and environmental well-being and duties of partnership on several public bodies allowed health concerns to legitimately appear on several policy agendas. This strengthened our role in local regeneration work and initiatives such as SureStart. Despite this welcome progress, the government has not given public health the same priority as illness services. Although promoting the idea that the

NHS must take more responsibility for health inequalities is welcome, policy to strengthen the public health infrastructure remains essential.

THE WORK

In 1997, in line with our developing philosophy, we gained the agreement of the chief executive to rename our department the Department of Social and Community Development. This more accurately reflected the work we were doing, and avoided the negative connotations which the term 'health promotion' had developed for some colleagues through being associated by successive governments with activity in primary medical care. Towards the end of the ten-year period under consideration, the departmental programme included:

- health needs assessment, identifying inequalities;
- developing health strategy in partnership with local people;
- developing policy to address inequalities, and ensuring policy informs resource allocation;
- ensuring services were effective, addressed inequality of access and fulfilled quality standards;
- work in partnership to ensure sustainable development;
- co-ordinating the authority's approach to area-based working and regeneration, including community development;
- co-ordinating the authority's work in involving the public and enabling a joint approach with other agencies;
- contributing to developing primary care.

These followed from the model we developed, and the work took place across all the identified levels, trying to embrace the principles we had agreed. A snapshot of work in 1997 is shown in Table 1.3.1. In practice work was focused on particular population groups, such as men, gay men, women, lesbians, children, young people, black and ethnic minority communities, people with disabilities, older adults and communities living in poverty. We also undertook disease-focused work to fulfil government policy, such as coronary heart disease, cancer prevention and HIV work. However, we tried to avoid a disease-based or settings-based approach, as it did not seem appropriate nor did it fit with our philosophy, and we feared it would divert attention from the root causes of ill health. As well as setting a health promotion agenda for others in the NHS, staff led on several areas of commissioning for the authority. All this work contributed to the development of our thinking, and gave us an opportunity to ensure all providers with whom we had a contract adhered to our principles and carried out certain annual objectives. Over time these became quite sophisticated, and included work to address poverty and environmental issues as well as a more traditional focus on providing health education as part of clinical work. Trusts did not receive extra money for this: they were expected to deliver as part of their contracted activity. We had few problems gaining agreement, though the work itself was inevitably mixed, with some delivering much more than the requirement and others much less.

Each Trust had a member of our staff assigned to them to support and develop their work, and this proved essential.

Alongside a health authority reorganization, we restructured our department into three teams – primary care, poverty and discrimination – with the aim of concentrating on the root causes of ill health. This arrangement helped to focus our thinking and activity in these areas. In the late 1990s we worked with officers from Sheffield City Council in developing a new approach called Area Action to the diverse areas of the city. The health authority, city council and community health services' trust had a director and senior officer attached to each area, who liaised with the council area panels and worked with local people. Four deprived areas were agreed as the highest priority and we provided a member of staff to each area, particularly to help in securing regeneration funds such as the Single Regeneration Budget, SureStart, Education Action Zone, On Track, and New Deal for Communities. This innovative work assisted several areas in gaining significant resources, developing strong area forums, and enabling greater local participation in policy and planning.

Each staff member in the departmental team had a portfolio of work, an area role, a role in commissioning and a responsibility for a health issue or a population group. Some also had a management role. Our staff came from a range of backgrounds, including nursing, teaching, social sciences and environmental work. Many had postgraduate qualifications in health promotion. The skills available in the department included community development, advocacy, participatory approaches, management of change, organization development, project management, facilitation, training, policy analysis, strategic planning, brokering and negotiation, all of which were applied to a social model of health. Staff went through programmes of personal development to acquire and sustain these skills.

Table 1.3.1 below gives a snapshot of work ongoing in 1997, and other examples are reported elsewhere in this book (see Greig and Parry's contribution and that of Standish, this volume).

Population group work	Health issues	Policy and planning	
			Table 1.3.1 A snapshot of work of the department in 1997
Black and ethnic minorities	Transport	Acute sector development	
Women, including pregnant women	Housing	Community and primary care sector development	
Men	Sexual health	Area based work in 12	
Children	Substance abuse	areas of the city	
Young people	Nutrition	Strategic partnership	
Older people	Accident prevention	development to increase	
Carers	Mental health	well-being in the city	
Travellers			
People with disabilities			
People with certain conditions, e.g. HIV, asthma			

Note: Work was generally a matrix of the above areas of action. For example, nutrition work related to several population groups and various geographical areas, and we undertook reviews to improve dietetic and nutrition services.

Apart from our work to support Healthy Sheffield and the establishment of the Area Action initiative, we also worked to influence citywide strategy. The health authority was a key partner in Sheffield First, a strategic group of chief executives, senior business people and elected councillors. A strategy to regenerate Sheffield was developed, with a member of our team seconded to support this, in particular the aspects relating to community development. We gradually became influential in city planning and ensuing action, and argued successfully for the social and economic strategies to be combined.

CONSTRAINTS

Inevitably, not all was plain sailing. Over the years we encountered a range of problems. Perhaps the biggest was the size of the agenda – it was hard to set clear priorities with so much need. The workload was huge, though some of this was of our own making. Resources were a further problem. During this period Sheffield was in a difficult financial state and no local organization had many resources for development. We had to be creative with what was a very small budget. The health promotion unit in the city council, with which we worked very closely, closed due to staff cuts in the early 1990s, and we also lost a number of our own staff who, due to tight budgets, were not replaced.

In some cases particular people opposed or blocked our activities, sometimes due to their own competing interests and in some cases because there was a lack of understanding of our approach. In addition, Sheffield's health authority was a demanding workplace, with a 'cutting edge' ethos – and we tended to make it more so. While our approach gave us a broad remit, there were inevitable tensions between departments which made for a sometimes stressful environment.

CONCLUSION

This has been a brief overview of the work of Sheffield's health promotion department over a ten-year period. Despite a hostile political climate and severe financial constraints for much of this time, we were still able to take forward radical work. We influenced local policy and services, enhanced Sheffield's bid for Health Action Zone status and for WHO status for the Healthy Sheffield initiative. We feel that clear objectives together with an explicit approach based on sound principles and linked to an evidence base helped us gain support from both the NHS and the local authority. Our approach remains valid today and we believe there is plenty of potential for others working in the statutory sector to go further than is perhaps realized in developing a radical agenda.

Looking back, there are a number of lessons which we would draw from all of this. First, a critical mass of health promotion specialists is necessary, drawn from a broad base of disciplines and skills. Second, to gain the benefits of this diversity it is crucial that staff share core values and beliefs. Time must be taken to develop a shared approach, and this may require protected 'time out'. Third, although the dedication, commitment and capability of staff enriched discussions and enabled a strong model to emerge, a lot still depended on personalities – both within the department and in positions of power.

The strength of partnership working and the resultant ability to influence agendas, funding and outcomes, speak for themselves. It is ironic that while the political climate has changed, and the rhetoric of partnership and promoting health is mainstream, pursuing a radical programme of work feels just as difficult now as it did in the early 1990s. Even in an apparently supportive political environment it may be hard to hold onto a clear and principled vision.

ACKNOWLEDGEMENTS

We are grateful to the all staff of Social and Community Development at Sheffield Health, who made this work possible.

2

SUSTAINABLE DEVELOPMENT AND HEALTH

Charles Secrett and Simon Bullock

SUSTAINABLE DEVELOPMENT: WHAT A GLOBAL PERSPECTIVE MEANS FOR THE UK

Following from the first Earth Summit, held in Rio de Janeiro in 1992, the most commonly accepted definition of sustainable development is 'development which meets the needs of the present, without compromising the ability of future generations to meet their own needs' (World Commission on Environment and Development, 1987). This means raising living standards and improving quality of life for all – not just the privileged. It means eradicating absolute poverty, where people are unable to meet their basic everyday needs. It means providing decent health care, and the physical and mental circumstances which allow individuals and communities to lead healthy and fulfilling lives. And it means doing so without exceeding environmental limits or using more ecological services than nature can regenerate, because both present and future generations need the flow of irreplaceable economic and social goods, services and other advantages from these ecological systems.

Given the state of the world, this is a major challenge. But these ambitious goals can be achieved if we are able to translate the requirements for sustainability into practical tools for policy-makers, and if sufficient political will can be mustered because humanity has the technological capacity, money, imagination and people power to make it happen. Governments are starting to address this challenge. For example, the UK government's sustainable development strategy (DETR, 1999b) says that the above definition means meeting four objectives at the same time:

- social progress which meets the needs of everyone;
- effective protection of the environment;
- prudent use of natural resources;
- maintenance of high and stable levels of economic growth and employment.

This is a useful framework, but the meanings of terms such as 'social progress', 'effective protection', 'prudent use' and 'stable levels of economic growth' need to be clearly defined for them to be useful in practical terms. The best starting point is to assess the limits of the planet's environmental systems, which provide irreplaceable life support functions alongside a range of natural products and services. These limits set a finite context in which development activities can occur, in order to avoid causing adverse environmental impacts and related economic or social problems – including public health problems. So, for any ecosystem, only so many natural resources can be taken out over a given period of time, or polluting substances put in, before its tolerance limits are exceeded and disruption occurs.

Global climate change is a clear example. The planet's atmosphere is capable of absorbing a certain amount of carbon dioxide (or other greenhouse gases) without destabilizing climate systems and weather patterns. But if carbon dioxide levels become too high, climate changes will occur. Beyond a certain temperature, precipitation or radiation impacts will occur which are beyond the capacity of species and ecosystems to tolerate. The scientific consensus of the Intergovernmental Panel on Climate Change is that carbon emissions from burning fossil fuels are already having a discernible impact on the climate, and global emissions of carbon dioxide should be reduced by at least 50 per cent by 2050 to avoid dangerous climate destabilization. This an example of an environmental limit, which helps us define 'effective protection of the environment' and 'prudent use of natural resources'.

Our bodies also have their own natural tolerance. Our metabolism can absorb only so much pollution before disease or death occurs. The problems of exposure to environmental insults, such as pesticides, hormone-mimicking chemicals, nuclear radiation, traffic pollution or other toxins, have demonstrated that maintaining high quality public health should set another powerful limit to damaging economic development activity.

If development is to be sustainable in ecosystem and human terms, policy options must be constrained not only by these environmental and health limits, but also by the sustainability requirement to ensure that *all* people are able to meet their needs in the present and the future. As available environmental resources are often limited, distribution of these resources will become a critical political issue. To achieve the sustainable development aim of 'social progress which recognizes the needs of everyone' means that development here must not undermine the needs of people in other countries. All countries should have access to their *fair share* of the earth's available resources – its natural goods as well as environmental services, like a stable climate – and this is not the case at present (see Figure 2.1).

These two concepts of 'environmental limits' and 'fair shares' of the earth's resources can be combined as a single idea, known as 'environmental space', to produce practical targets for policy-makers in every sector which show what individual countries must do to achieve sustainable development. Friends of the Earth, in association with the Wuppertal Institute in Germany, originated the concept of environmental space to calculate targets for countries throughout the world, explain how they can be met, and describe the sustainability benefits in social, economic and environmental terms (Carley and Spapens, 1998; McLaren et al., 1998).

To take climate change as an illustration, Britain emits 500 million tonnes of carbon dioxide (the main greenhouse gas) annually, equivalent to just under 10 tonnes per person. Globally, over 20 billion tonnes are emitted annually by 5.5 billion people, an average of around 4 tonnes each. By 2050, when the world's

Figure 2.1   Per capita carbon dioxide emissions for different countries in 2000

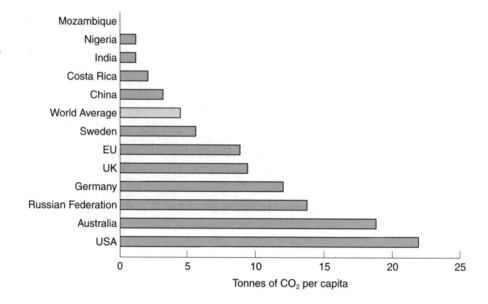

Figure 2.1   Per capita carbon dioxide emissions for different countries in 2000

population will be 10 billion, global greenhouse gas emissions must be reduced by at least half to stabilize our changing climate, so a fair share of climate space will allow just one tonne of carbon dioxide emission per person. To reach this target, Britain will have had to reduce its carbon dioxide emissions by 90 per cent from current levels. Similar targets can be calculated for our use of other natural resources, such as virgin timber, water, aluminium and steel. These are summarized in Table 2.1, while the basis on which these calculations are made is explained more fully in a series of on-line resources.[1]

Table 2.1
Sustainability targets for the UK, by 2050

Environmental resource used	Target reduction by 2050 (%)
carbon dioxide	88
virgin aluminium	88
virgin timber	73
iron ore	83
water	15
global agricultural land[2]	27
chlorine	100

These targets provide a UK context for determining the necessary actions to achieve sustainable development. They show the amount of environmental resources available to the UK to achieve 'social progress which recognizes the needs of everyone'. It is important to stress that sustainability policies based on these targets do not imply mass redundancies, increased poverty or economic collapse. These pollution and resource use reductions can be achieved with already available technologies by, for example, hugely increasing the efficient use of natural resources by ten times or more (McLaren et al., 1998; von Weisacker, et al., 1997). But it does require that our economy is harnessed far more to meeting people's needs efficiently, rather than simply to increasing economic growth, waste and pollution without respect for sustainability limits, and then somehow trying to mitigate the adverse environmental and social consequences.[3] A higher priority for public health goals is therefore a key element in ensuring that government policies are focused on social progress for all.

MEETING NEEDS IN THE UK

'Social progress which recognizes the needs of all people' effectively means that, as a minimum, certain basic needs are met for all. Box 2.1 shows a 'charter' of such basic health needs, published by the Public Health Alliance (now the UK Public Health Association).

BOX 2.1   THE BASIS FOR HEALTH FOR ALL PEOPLE

Income which provides the material means to remain healthy.
Homes that are safe, warm, dry, secure and affordable.
Food that is safe, nourishing, widely available and affordable.
Transport that permits accessible, safe travel at reasonable cost and encourages fuel economy and a clean environment.
Work that is properly rewarded, within or outside of the home, which is worthwhile and free from hazards to health and safety.
Environments which are protected from dangerous pollution and radiation, and planned to preserve and enhance our quality of life.
Public services which provide care for those in need, and support for carers; clean, safe water and waste disposal; adequate childcare and recreation facilities.
Education and information which give all the necessary information to keep us healthy, and the confidence and resources to tackle the causes of ill health.
Comprehensive health services properly resourced, free at the point of use and sensitive to our health needs.
Equal opportunity to good health regardless of class, race, gender, physical ability, age or sexual orientation.
Security which gives freedom from war, and from the threats of crime and violence.
Social policy which recognises the importance of self-fulfilment and supportive social relationships, and promotes these through the provision of domiciliary support and other services.

(The Charter for Public Health, published by the
Public Health Alliance, 1988.)

This is a key link between the public health and environmental movements: the social aims of sustainable development mean that in a world of limited environmental resources, basic needs – public health goals – need to be prioritized. As a mechanism to achieve this, granting citizens statutory rights to a clean and healthy environment, pure water, clean air, uncontaminated land, wholesome food, and peace and quiet, would give a constitutional guarantee for everyone, whatever their social or professional standing, that the state recognizes the fundamental importance of sustainable development, and strives to achieve environmental and human health.

Policy changes

As a first step, sustainability strategies must assess which individuals and communities are lacking these prerequisites for good health. Britain's track record is patchy, to say the least. Progress has been made in some areas, such as housing, with government support for the Warm Homes Bill in 2000, and action by some health authorities on energy efficiency projects as preventative health measures. But in many other major areas, such as eradicating food poverty, ensuring access to decent transport and minimizing environmental pollution, deep problems remain. Poorer people suffer most from these problems, as research by FoE and others has shown (Boardman et al., 1999; Friends of the Earth, 2001). Despite the sustainable development plan, there is still no coherent, integrated strategy coordinated by the UK government to tackle these problems. Yet it is a fundamental requirement of sustainable development that such inequities and unmet basic needs are resolved as the highest social priority.

We elect governments to set the rules by which we play the game of public life. Government has five main instruments – policy, regulation, taxes, expenditure and education – to foster sustainable behaviour throughout society. It must take more opportunities to ensure that basic needs are met in a way which also meets broader, global environmental imperatives. So, for example, policies should be co-ordinated and integrated on an inter-departmental basis, and promote sustainability objectives; regulation and policy targets should be based on precautionary environmental and human health requirements; taxation should discourage unsustainable polluting and inefficient resource-use activities in business and household consumption, while encouraging sustainable activities; and expenditure should be targeted towards helping the poorest improve their quality of life, while providing nationwide infrastructure and services, such as waste minimization, resource conservation, public transport and energy efficiency.

The government could promote such joined-up thinking and action by sponsoring inter-departmental legislation based on delivering sustainability goals rather than perpetuating departmental competition for legislative time which invariably leads to disconnected policies and missed opportunities to integrate environmental, social and economic objectives. The 'green ministers' group from each department could prioritize this type of coordination and help spread best practice across government. Currently, 'compartmentalization' is still a problem, and public health and environmental issues – which do affect more than one department – are not properly integrated across government. Yet if these initiatives happen, people are more likely to be both more motivated and better able to respond to public education programmes which exhort 'everyone to do their bit for the environment'.

As well as assessing and dealing with existing problems, sustainability policies in all sectors should include both strategic and operational assessments of their distributional impacts. Environmental Impact Assessment (EIA) has been in the policy-makers' tool-box for some time, but what is needed is a joined-up consideration of policies for their separate and combined health, environmental and distributional impacts. One of the main recommendations of the Acheson Inquiry into Inequalities in Health was that 'all policies likely to have a direct or indirect effect on health should be evaluated in terms of their impact on health inequalities, and should be formulated in such a way that by favouring the less well off they will, wherever possible, reduce such inequalities' (Acheson, 1998). The need for Health Impact Assessments (HIAs) is written into the public health strategies of all four nations of the UK, and HIAs should link with EIAs to address equity assessments.

One key policy change needed is to change the burden of proof for potentially health-damaging activities. As in many other sectors, the precautionary principle should apply here. For example, chemicals policy deals with uncertainty and risk by allowing chemicals to be dispersed into the environment or used in consumer products until a danger to people's health is proven, but there are severe drawbacks in taking this approach (see Box 2.2).

BOX 2.2   DANGEROUS CHEMICALS?

Only 14 per cent of high volume chemicals (over 1,000 tonnes/year produced in the EU) have the minimum set of basic safety data.
21 per cent of high volume chemicals have no safety data at all.
Only 30 per cent of high volume chemicals have minimal information on whether they accumulate in our bodies.
There is even less known about lower volume chemicals.

(Allanou et al., 1999)

This presumption of innocence should not continue where synthetic chemicals are concerned. Some 60,000 already exist, and over 2,000 new ones enter the market place every year. These chemicals end up in the environment, and in our bodies, so clearly, policy-makers must ensure that they are safe. The current approach does not do so, and imposes unsustainable health pressures on present and future generations. Children, in particular, are at risk from dangerous chemical pollutants (Friends of the Earth, 1998). As a first corrective step, persistent and bio-accumulative chemicals – such as PCBs and dioxins – should be phased out. Equally importantly, the burden of proof in law should be changed so that manufacturers are required to demonstrate that their products are safe.

Those who put human well-being at risk should have to prove that any possible adverse impacts were not caused by their actions. Currently, those who suffer must prove cause and effect. This is extremely difficult, given the number of possible chemical, lifestyle or other potential causes of illness and the analytic task of identifying and measuring the effects of chronic, mixed exposures. Such a change would encourage the development of safer technologies and products. A further change needed to protect future generations is to replace the widespread use of narrow risk assessments as policy tools. Risk assessments traditionally ask whether a technology is 'safe' – taking into account exposures, toxicities, and a (political) interpretation of what level of risk is deemed 'acceptable', but this misses a range of complexities (see Box 2.3).

BOX 2.3   RISK ASSESSMENTS

Narrow risk assessments ignore complexities such as:
● effects we don't know about yet;
● how the effects interact with other environmental exposures;
● people have differing abilities to cope, and unique histories of exposure to hazards;
● all organisms are too complex to allow reliable prediction of effects.

They ignore questions about the activity such as:
● is this activity ethical?
● is the activity needed?
● are there less damaging ways of accomplishing the same purpose?

O'Brien (2000) argues that 'alternatives' assessment should replace 'risk assessment' – with risk assessment having a much smaller role to play in decision making.

Before deciding whether to pursue a particular technology or product development option, it would often be better if policy-makers were to question not only whether or not it is safe, but also whether it is the best way forward given sustainability goals. For example, in the context of genetically modified (GM) foods, instead of asking only 'Is GM food safe for people or does it harm the environment', policy-makers, farmers and consumers should also be asking questions such as 'What sort of agricultural system do we want?' GM crop technologies supplied by a very few companies, combined with patent controls over these products, have the potential to markedly alter both agricultural systems and farm and rural community demographics. The full implications of different development models need to be debated in public, rather than hidden in risk assessment models used by civil servants and ministers to decide among themselves what type of development should proceed. A participative and open political process requires considered and informed debate in which health professionals are actively engaged. This issue has been covered extensively by the Economic and Social Research Council (Stirling and Mayer, 1999).

WIN-WIN-WIN ISSUES

Public health needs should be met through development programmes that have minimal adverse environmental impacts. Even more so, the resolution of environmental problems such as contaminated land, polluted air or water, and unhealthy food or living conditions, is a prerequisite for improving public health. Unsurprisingly, preventative public health measures are usually the most effective methods for achieving these mutually supportive objectives, as the philosophy of 'prevention is better than cure' is synonymous with best practice in environmental protection. For example, one of the best ways to tackle many health problems caused by poor quality housing is to improve energy efficiency ratings, which also conserves resource use and reduces pollution: good for both people and environment. As energy conservation programmes create significant numbers of new jobs and help companies and householders save money by using less resources, they are also good for the economy. Policies and programmes which simultaneously achieve economic, health and environmental benefits have 'win-win-win' sustainability outcomes (Bullock, 1995). Sustainable development policies try to maximize such opportunities, and minimize the trade-offs between the different objectives. Examples of three other broad areas where public health and economic needs could be met far more directly and efficiently than at present, and with lower environmental impacts, are given below.

Local economic development

The Acheson Inquiry clearly identified differences in the health of unemployed and employed people (Acheson, 1998). It noted that employment is 'significant in providing purpose, income, social support, structure to life and a means of participating in society'. Many local environmental measures are particularly good at creating jobs, as well as delivering environmental and health benefits. Three examples are boosting energy efficiency measures in buildings, improving public transport and developing community waste minimization and reuse/recycling schemes. Such development activities all deliver more jobs per pound invested than less sustainable alternatives such as higher power/fuel purchases, more driving and road building, and landfilling or incinerating waste (Jenkins, 1994). These and other initiatives such as local food schemes (allotments, farmers' markets, community orchards and food co-ops), credit unions, LETS (local exchange trading schemes) and community self-build housing, demonstrate how environmentally sustainable economic activities can meet people's needs directly, with large public health and quality of life gains.

Most of these programmes do not operate nationally, although the benefits of replicating them throughout Britain would be significant. Nevertheless, some are expanding as their benefits become apparent. The most important economic catalyst increasing support for such schemes is likely to be their regenerative effects. Current community regeneration initiatives focus heavily on government grants and inward investment to pump money into poorer, disadvantaged areas, yet many economic problems remain – particularly the subsequent outflow of these funds from the communities affected. Sustainable development initiatives help keep money in the local area (Jenkins, 1994). For example, over 80 per cent of the money spent in supermarkets leaves the local economy in which the shop trades. Money spent in a farmers' market or through vegetable box schemes, which directly benefits local farmers and businesses, stays within the local economy, generating more local economic activity and jobs as a result. This 'multiplier' effect is an important reason why local authorities and regeneration professionals should prioritize these initiatives. The Social Exclusion Unit offers keeping money within neighbourhoods as one of its 'key ideas' in its strategy on Neighbourhood Renewal (Cabinet Office, 2000).

Housing

Fuel poverty – the inability to keep your home warm at reasonable cost – contributes to some 30,000 people dying prematurely every winter in Britain, simply because they are cold and damp. This is a major, and almost wholly avoidable, scandal: much colder countries like Sweden do not experience this phenomenon, because they insist on high energy efficiency and insulation ratings for buildings. From an environmental and social perspective, Britain's housing stock is in a bad way. The average energy efficiency rating for the whole stock is only 35 out of 100, where new houses average around 70. There are millions of houses which rate below 20 out of 100, and of course poor housing is largely occupied by the poor and the elderly.

Poor people, by definition, have the least to spend on fuel and suffer from living in homes which are the least efficient in converting fuel to warmth. The elderly are the most vulnerable to the effects of cold, damp living conditions. Nationwide measures to improve energy efficiency in the worst housing – along with increases in benefits and tackling some of the electricity and gas companies' more regressive charging policies – would have major public health benefits and reduce health inequalities. It will require co-ordinated intervention by many housing, poverty and environmental agencies, working together with the private sector, to improve this situation but it can be done. It is encouraging to see the pioneering efforts of some health authorities, such as Doncaster and Cornwall, which are investing in housing improvements specifically to prevent illness and so reduce future costs on primary care services. The passage of the Warm Homes Act 2000 mandates the government to eradicate fuel poverty by 2010.

Transport

Transport policies have obvious impacts on health. Over the past 30 years, transport policies have overwhelmingly favoured road over rail, and private over public transport. The result has been continuing high rates of death and serious injury due to road accidents, as well as a range of other health costs. The Department of Health estimates that urban air pollution, mainly caused by traffic, causes 12,000 to 24,000 premature deaths each year. Over 3,000 people are killed in road accidents each year, and a further 50,000 seriously injured. Noise pollution reduces quality of life, and heavy traffic severs communities. The lack of non-car transport options also adversely affects public health and quality of life. For example, from the early 1980s to the mid-1990s, a large network of out-of-town superstores aimed at car-driving consumers appeared, encouraged by favourable planning rules and new road building. This directly led to the closure of thousands of local and smaller shops, and gave us the modern phenomenon of 'food deserts' – areas where it is simply not possible to buy fresh, affordable, healthy food. This problem is so severe that the government's Social Exclusion Unit made the issue a priority area in 1998 (Department of Health, 2000c).

Economic development policies create serious environmental and social justice problems. Most households have access to a car, but while only 4 per cent of those in the richest fifth of the population lack access to a car, the figure is 70 per cent for the poorest fifth, who have to make do with other alternatives, if alternatives exist at all. Moreover, a significant minority of people – many elderly and disabled people, and all children – cannot use a car, and for them public transport services are crucial. Transport policies must be assessed for their distributional impact, because it is the poorest who suffer most from traffic pollution, noise, road accidents (children in social class V are five times more likely to be knocked down by a car than those in social class I), expensive or unavailable public transport and lack of access to facilities (Boardman et al., 1999). Priority must given to those who suffer the worst effects. A decent, sustainable transport system must ensure everyone has access to services which enable them to live healthy lives. We need policies and expenditures which prioritize convenient, clean and affordable public transport options, safe walking and cycling routes, and planning decisions which reduce the need to travel to access essential services.

AGENCIES FOR CHANGE

Achieving sustainability objectives in public health arenas will require many different groups of people to be involved and active, not merely the concerned and interested. While individual citizens can, of course, contribute solutions themselves, national government must be responsible for implementing critical changes through revised policies and programmes. Additionally, health professionals have opportunities to bring about change by, for example, lobbying for national sustainability policies and expenditures, giving individuals the information they need to make their own choices, or by changing local practices. The external actions of organization – such as health authorities' Health Action Zones – are discussed elsewhere in this book. Internal actions are reviewed briefly below.

Internal policies

Health professionals interested in promoting sustainable development can also improve the internal policies of the health service. The NHS is the biggest employer in Europe and causes major, mostly adverse, environmental impacts through its transport, waste disposal, energy use and food sourcing activities. There are many opportunities for the NHS to improve its own poor sustainability performance. For example, health services could locate hospitals in places near to population centres to reduce the need to travel, use high-efficiency micro-power (CHP) plants for energy generation, minimize driving and purchase efficient and cleaner-fuelled vehicles, increase recycling, reuse and waste minimization, and source local and organic food. All health authorities and health care providers should have strong environmental policies. Of course, there are financial benefits too, for example, energy efficiency and reduced waste strategies will save scarce health care resources.

Health authorities and health professionals need to be aware of the external policy agenda and be prepared to shape it. Environmental tax reforms are now a major part of each government budget announcement. In April 2001, the climate change levy came into force, which increases energy costs for businesses, and recycles the money back through reduced National Insurance contributions. This levy is a part of an increasing trend to increase taxes on environmental 'bads' (such as fossil fuel use, waste disposal, pollution) while decreasing it on 'goods' (such as income or employment). Some sectors gain or lose more than others, for example, labour-intensive sectors will do well, as reduced National Insurance contributions will give them more benefits than costs from increases in energy spending. The NHS is a major potential winner here as, compared with other sectors, energy spending is a far smaller part of its budget than staffing costs. Modelling the effects of a modest carbon tax, with revenues recycled in lower National Insurance contributions, puts the employment gains for the health/social sector at 27,000 by 2010 (Cambridge Econometrics, 1998). But to date lobbying against environmental tax reform by those who may lose out is far more organized than lobbying for such changes by those who stand to gain.

KEY CHALLENGES FOR THE FUTURE

One of the starkest sustainability challenges confronting present and future generations is the scale, intensity and rate of climatic change which is expected over coming decades as a result of human activity. Already we can see the potential, and perhaps reality, of the environmental and human health threats that climatic disruption poses, including the increased incidence of catastrophic extreme weather events, such as the hurricanes that battered Central America and south-east Africa in 1998 and 1999; seasonal floods and droughts, which hit the United States, China and central Asia between 1997 and 2000; changing vectors for insect- or animal-borne diseases, such as malaria or Nile Fever; and rising sea levels inundating small island states and heavily populated coastal zones. Stopping dangerous climate change is one of the biggest global health challenges facing us. But keeping climate change in check has major implications for countries like the UK, which currently uses large quantities of fossil fuel. There is real potential for the public health and environmental sectors to join forces and advocate the necessary changes. A healthy home is best achieved through high levels of energy efficiency; a healthy transport system is organized around walking, cycling and public transport. Healthy food comes from less intensive farming. There are major environmental benefits from well-designed public health strategies. These benefits work both ways. Protecting our planet's ecosystem is an essential condition for long-term public health.

NOTES

1 Summary briefings are available on energy, land, water, metals and wood, at: http://www.foe.co.uk/campaigns/sustainable_development/publications/tworld/briefs.html

2 Currently, the UK uses an agricultural area of 17 million hectares, and is a net 'importer' of a further 4.1 million hectares – land in other countries which is used to grow food for consumption in the UK. A fair share approach to available agricultural land implies that the UK should be a 'net exporter' of around 2 million hectares of land.

3 Economic success is traditionally defined by governments as growth in Gross Domestic Product. But this takes no account of what sort of economic activity is generated. If economic growth is obtained at the expense of the environment or people's health and quality of life, then it is neither sustainable nor worth sustaining. See: http://www.foe.co.uk/campaigns/sustainable_development/progress/annex1.htm

2.1

FOOD AND HEALTH: NATIONAL AND INTERNATIONAL POLICY PERSPECTIVES

Martin Caraher

Our lives are all touched – inevitably – by food. Much research has used food as a metaphor to explore, for example, family relationships, gender, age or ethnicity (Brannen et al., 1994), and food has also been taken as a measure of globalization and the power of large companies (Ritzer, 2000). Yet health promotion has largely ignored wider elements of the food system – including issues of ecology and sustainability – opting instead for an approach based on the provision of nutrition and dietary advice. Many local health promotion food projects have a radical philosophy but are operating against a range of global forces (McGlone et al., 1999). This chapter explores the national and international dimensions of food policy, and argues that health promoters must focus their efforts 'upstream' on the determinants of food supply, facing up to the global nature of food production.

GLOBALIZATION, HEALTH AND FOOD

As Murcott (1999) notes, you can 'search in vain' for literature on social movements that aim to influence food policy. The food industry is one of the main influences on consumers, yet health promotion has taken the easy option of working with capital, by helping to turn citizens into consumers of healthy eating and nutrition advice (Grace, 1991; Lupton, 1994, 1996), and ignoring the role of structural factors on food choice and nutrition. Like their communicable counterparts, non-communicable diseases cross borders too but in different ways. While the former usually spread by infection, the latter spread through lifestyle and social changes (Drewnoski and Popkin, 1997). There is no doubt that in the 'First World' we eat a different and better diet than our predecessors 100 years ago. We live longer, are taller and do not suffer diseases of deprivation associated with food. But more of us than ever are affected by food-related diseases such as heart disease and cancer, more of us are obese and there is still food poverty in our societies (Acheson, 1998; Dobson, 1997; Dobson et al., 1994; Leather, 1996).

Globalization has a number of meanings. For our purposes, the first refers to the economic process of trade liberalization of food markets. Globalization also has cultural and ideological dimensions, sometimes referred to as

'McDonaldization' or 'Coca-Colaization' (Prendergrast, 1993; Ritzer, 2000). People are being encouraged to think of food and drink as coming, not from farmers or the earth, but from giant corporations (Klein, 2000). A recent opinion poll found that 65 per cent of people in China recognize the brand name of Coca-Cola, 42 per cent recognize Pepsi and 40 per cent recognize Nestlé (Gallup, 1995). This is the result of a methodical moulding of taste, with the large corporations, controlling production and distribution chains, now the primary drivers in dietary change. The scale and pace of globalization are being accelerated by new technologies and falling global trade barriers. The global trade liberalization advanced by the World Trade Organisation (WTO) is allowing rich consumer societies to adopt a diet produced globally. The corollary is that developing countries, with cheap land and labour, are encouraged to grow food for the global market, resulting in the demise of agriculture for local needs – with the result that at the height of the 1984 Ethiopian famine, green beans were still being exported to UK supermarkets (Athanasiou, 1996). The neo-liberal economic rationale is that the income from such trade enables people to buy food, but cheap food for the consumer in the developed world may not square with fair prices for the producer (see Box 2.1.1).

BOX 2.1.1   WORLD BANANA TRADE

Three trans-national companies control 80 per cent of the world banana trade with:
2 per cent of the retail price of a banana going to the fieldworker;
5 per cent to the farmer;
88 per cent to food chain intermediaries such as the importer, wholesaler, freight company and retailer.

(Based on Paxton, 1994)

The globalization of food production has other adverse health effects. The distance food travels – the 'food miles' – between producer and consumer rose by a third in 15 years at the end of the twentieth century (Paxton, 1994). This increase in food miles is associated with increasing use of pesticides and packaging, and transport pollution. These costs are not passed directly to the consumer, but fall on communities, the health service and the environment (see box 2.1.2).

BOX 2.1.2   FOOD MILES TRAVELLED IN EUROPE AND THE USA

The average European weekend shopping trolley contains goods that have already travelled 4,000 km before we take them home. In the US, one study calculated each item in the trolley travels an average of 2,000 km between grower and consumer.

(Clunies-Ross and Hildyard, 1992)

FOOD SAFETY AND FOOD SECURITY

In many developed countries, the big food scandal is not food safety but food poverty, with people either going hungry or being unable to afford nutritionally sound diets (Dobson et al., 1994). Food security – the right of individuals and communities to an adequate, culturally appropriate diet – is the neglected issue in food policy. The Food and Agriculture Organisation (FAO, 1999) estimates that for the period 1995–97, up to 790 million people in the developing world did not have enough to eat. But the same report points out that in the industrialized countries of the First World there were an additional 8 million people under-nourished and suffering serious food deprivation.

The food poverty we see today in developed countries is different from that of a century ago. Then, some sections of society simply did not have the means to buy or cook food, creating well-documented health inequality between the 'haves' and the 'have nots'. The current situation is one of relative rather than absolute poverty, as table 2.1.1 illustrates (Dobson 1997; Dowler, 1998, 1999). In developed economies, such as the UK, the poverty gap is also a cultural one and food is one way that people can feel isolated from the cultural mainstream: a family may be well nourished nutritionally but still experience deprivation through lack of access to valued foods, preferred foods or consistent amounts of food (Crotty, 1999).

Table 2.1.1 The new inequalities?

The old food poverty	The new food poverty
Lack of food	Overabundance of processed foods
Under-nutrition	Lack of balance
Cost of food	Relative cost of food
Removal from the norm	Socially and culturally isolated

THE NEW FOOD (IN)SECURITY

The emergence of 'food deserts' is one example of the new food poverty and the need for a shift in emphasis from approaches to food and nutrition based on knowledge and skills to one based on access and resources (Caraher et al., 1998; Lang and Caraher, 1998). The term 'food deserts' describes the idea that in an affluent country like the UK there are many areas where cheap and healthy food is simply not available. In the UK food retailing is dominated by a few large companies: by the end of the 1990s five food retailers (Sainsbury, Tesco, Safeway, Asda and Gateway) accounted for 70 per cent of the total UK grocery market. This concentration of market share was accompanied by the development of out-of-town supermarkets – 'Cathedrals of Consumption' (Fine, 1993) – and the closure of large numbers of local shops. The result contributed to the demise of inner cities, the destruction of rural economies and the creation of food deserts with the physical and social isolation of single mothers, the elderly and those without access to a car or public transport, among others. The concentration of food retailing in this way is not confined to the UK: Hungary had over 5000 supermarkets and hyper-markets in 1997, and the seven in Poland in 1995 were expected to grow to 70 by 2001.

FOOD POLICY: THE WAY FORWARD FOR HEALTH PROMOTION

Food policy embraces all those policies affecting food and the food economy. As well as food supply, it also includes policies not directly concerned with health such as transport and planning laws (OECD, 1981). Food policy is multifaceted and inter-professional in scope and has to engage with issues such as the emerging global marketplace and international laws and regulations governing food trade. Government health promotion policy in relation to food continues to focus on the transfer of knowledge and skills, and encourages behavioural interventions rather than addressing structural factors. This is a shame, since there is ample evidence that people already possess the skills and knowledge, but not always the resources necessary to put their intentions into action (Charles and Kerr, 1986; Lang et al., 1999).

To successfully tackle the issues raised above, in the interests of health, would require health promotion workers not just to have a radically different approach but also new skills and a professional influence backed by wider social forces. Tactically, health educators and promoters could take the opportunity to move away from an emphasis on consumers and to build on the experience of alliances; but alliances that end up subordinating health promotion to commercial interests should obviously be avoided. Currently, we need more evidence of the health gain, if any, that results from alliances between commercial companies, such as supermarkets, and the health promotion agencies which focus on the provision of health information for consumers.

HEALTH PROMOTION POLICY RESPONSES

One example of a comprehensive regional analysis and clear policy response comes from Scotland where the Foodworks Enquiry noted: 'Essentially the problem is that Scotland has minimal control of its food supply and that its food choices, national and individual, are principally determined by interests for whom the health and prosperity of Scotland's people are not their main concerns' (Foodworks Enquiry, 1997). The enquiry concluded:

> Whilst community action is essential in defining health needs, in controlling the excesses of food market operations at the local level and in demonstrating the benefits of alternative approaches to improving the Scottish diet, only government action can provide the framework within which substantive improvements to the Scottish diet and to the ability of people living on low incomes to exercise healthy food choices can be developed.

Many projects using community development approaches are based on an assumption of inadequate personal resources (Lang and Caraher, 1998; McGlone et al., 1999; UNICEF, 1994). In concentrating on communities which already have identified problems, there is the risk of imposing an extra, unsustainable, burden. While such projects may improve self-esteem, engender a sense of empowerment, and provide knowledge and skills, where do people go with these? I argue that unless the determinants of poor health, at global, national and regional levels, are tackled, community development will just continue to 'pick up the pieces'. In developing 'upstream' approaches, health promoters must address food policy and a number of regional and national examples provide hope here, including the Knoxville Food Policy Council in the USA, the Toronto Food Policy Council in Canada and Norway's national food and nutrition policy (Baum, 1998; Dahlberg, 1992). In addition, the International Conference on Nutrition provides an example of global commitment, requiring national governments to monitor the food security of 'at risk' social groups (FAO/WHO, 1992).

Experience from the Toronto Food Policy Council (Welsh and MacRae, 1998) and other such initiatives suggests that approaches to food insecurity based on anti-hunger advocacy or on the rights of consumers does not challenge the food system or its economic logic. Using their ideas, the following list is offered as an audit tool for all food projects – whether local, regional or national.

1   Projects should not use strategies based on charity. Charity can be destructive in the way it depoliticizes hunger and poverty, and the way it divides us as full participants in society.
2   Health professionals, especially health promotion specialists, dieticians and nutritionists, can play an important role in food advocacy.
3   Projects should explicitly address the deskilling involved in the globalization process. Projects should seek to reskill, not just counsel or educate about consumer choices. Skill development involves not only food-related practices, but also understanding the systems in one's community, and gaining a sense of being able to manoeuvre within them – or even change them.
4   Food projects must plan to solve multiple problems at once. Since community food insecurity is the result of a number of factors, it makes little sense to address only one element at a time. Projects should address some combination of access to resources, price, physical accessibility, and quality of food.
5   Projects should deliberately take back some degree of control of food distribution from the dominant food system and re-invest in distribution through community and public spaces – schools, community facilities, social housing complexes, health centres, and so on.

The evolution of food policy has been left to the market for too long, and the influence of public health thinking has been negligible (Lang, 1999). The result has been the 'invisible hand of the market' dominating public policy on population food security. To be effective, health promoters must confront these powerful interests with the aim of creating local and regional sustainable food economies based on a mix of what is best about globalization and the local situation. The riots during the WTO negotiations in Seattle in 1999 demonstrated the concern of the public on food issues (Sinclair, 2000). Now health promoters must find some way to give voice to people – locally and globally – in their concerns over the future of food and the globalization process. The World Health Organisation's food and nutrition action plan (World Health Organisation, 2000) outlines a way to move from food growing to food policy influence and may offer a blueprint for health promotion practice.

2.2

LOCAL COMMUNITIES AND SUSTAINABLE REGENERATION IN THE EAST END OF SHEFFIELD

Sue Greig and Neil Parry

Following the collapse of employment in the steel and engineering industries, Sheffield's East End has seen considerable physical regeneration and economic development over the past 15 years. But despite this, the experience of local communities is one of deepening economic, social and environmental decline. The electoral ward of Darnall is one of only three in the city where mortality rates under 75 years have significantly worsened over the last 15 years, compared with England and Wales (Richardson, 1999). The area has the highest death rates from coronary heart disease in the city and hospital admissions for respiratory disease are well above the city average.

Yet in the East End of Sheffield prosperity and deprivation sit side by side. The area provides over a quarter of the jobs in the Sheffield travel-to-work area, but local communities, particularly those of black and minority ethnic origin, have some of the highest rates of unemployment (about 40 per cent) in the city (Herzmark, 1997). Customers from more affluent areas travel – mostly by private car – to the East End's many sports, leisure and retail facilities, past run-down public parks and impoverished local amenities. The consequence of such traffic-generating leisure and retail development is air quality which consistently fails the standards set to protect health. The designation of the East End as an 'air quality management area', followed by action to improve air quality, is now a legal requirement (DETR, 1999a). For local communities the legacy of the East End's 'economic revival' has been increasing poverty, social exclusion and environmental degradation, and for the city as a whole, widening inequalities in health. Sustainable development requires new thinking about urban regeneration, moving away from the old language of 'trade-offs' and towards approaches which deliver environmental sustainability, economic prosperity and social inclusion *all at the same time* (DETR, 2000a).

TINSLEY COMMUNITY HEALTH AND TRANSPORT PROJECT (1997-99)

In November 1997 a community development project was established in Tinsley, a small community of 4,000 residents in Sheffield's East End, cut off from the rest of Sheffield by the M1 motorway. The project was a response to a wide consultation on transport and health issues conducted by an inter-agency group over the previous year, which had highlighted a lack of local participation in transport and land use planning decisions with major impacts on health and well-being (Sheffield and Rotherham Transport and Health Group, 1996, 1997). Tinsley Community Forum, a well-established and respected group, had been campaigning for many years on the damaging impact of high traffic levels, noise, and air pollution on quality of life in their community.

The community health and transport project had two clear and interrelated aims: first, to put the Tinsley community at the centre of decision-making processes about transport, planning and development policies which affect quality of life in their neighbourhood; and second, to develop more 'joined-up' policy-making, by giving more weight to social and environmental considerations in future policies for the area. The project ran for two years and had considerable success in raising the profile of the issues facing Tinsley residents, promoting discussion and debate between local people and senior policy-makers, and galvanizing the local authorities to work collaboratively on the social, economic and environmental issues affecting Tinsley.

A two-stage evaluation of the project was completed through semi-structured interviews with project steering group members and other key players, undertaken halfway through and again at the end of the project (East End Quality of Life, 2000a). Those interviewed pointed to a range of factors felt to be key ingredients of the project's success, including a tenacious project worker with campaigning and negotiating skills developed within the trade union movement; a strong local infrastructure with transport and health issues already high on the community's agenda; and some prior ownership of the project and commitment to it from statutory agencies, in particular local public health, social and community development, environmental protection and area regeneration/social inclusion departments, as a result of previous inter-agency working on transport and health.

In addition, the use of innovative approaches to community engagement was seen to be important. For example, a theatre group was commissioned to work with Tinsley Forum on a sketch of 'Life in Tinsley', performed at the community launch of the project. This proved an extremely effective and affirming way of engaging the hearts and minds of an invited panel of local and health authority representatives, as well as the wider community audience. Similarly, the project made effective use of the media. A 'Tinsley Millennium Man' in white overalls, large black respirator, ear defenders and oxygen tanks posed the question 'Is this the future? Do we do something about the pollution now or will we have to use respirators, etc. to protect our health in the future?' Coupled with statistics on respiratory disease for the local area, this captured the interest of national and local TV and press, resulting in some sympathetic and thoughtful coverage (see Box 2.2.1). The project also monitored nitrogen dioxide levels at five back garden sites in Tinsley, from 1998 onwards, giving the community forum direct access to its own data on air quality. The area now has a group of community activists who are well versed in air quality standards and legislation, and the extent to which these are being breached in their own neighbourhood.

> ## BOX 2.2.1 TWO SIDES
>
> Both sides of the motorway will soon be further developed ... It will be a tremendous boost in terms of facilities and tourism throughout South Yorkshire – unless you happen to live there ... At Tinsley, the prospect of a string of world class projects fail to generate any enthusiasm whatsoever among many local people. Noise and air pollution represent a legitimate concern, with hospital admissions for asthma three times the average ... It's easy to congratulate ourselves on winning large-scale development and luring business into the city; but we can't afford to ignore the significant social impact that changing the face of Sheffield is bringing.
>
> (*Sheffield Telegraph*, 20 February 1998)

As well as these successes, the evaluation highlighted a number of challenges, inherent in the project's ambitious aims, to which we now turn.

COMMUNITY AND ORGANIZATIONAL DEVELOPMENT: THE SLOW PACE OF CHANGE

It is difficult and time-consuming to support a demoralized community and a hard-pressed group of community activists, meet the demands of bureaucratic regeneration-funding regimes, engage with the issues, participate in decision and debate, and have faith that action will follow.

The project played a significant role as a 'broker' facilitating communication between sections of different public authorities that might otherwise have remained stubbornly in their 'professional silos'. For example, the project instigated a seminar on 'planning and sustainability' which brought together strategic, area and development control planners with community representatives. This was influential in stimulating debate on how local planning procedures might constructively respond to the challenge of sustainable development. Of course, 'joined-up' working requires organizational cultures to change and new working relationships to be built, and this takes time, with many setbacks along the way.

PARTNERSHIP WORKING – MORE TALK, LESS ACTION?

Local communities in the East End now have regular access to senior policymakers through the 'East End strategy group' where representatives from public health, environmental protection, planning, transportation and regeneration meet regularly with community and voluntary sector representatives. The guiding principle of this group is to work towards a vision of environmental, social and economic sustainability for Sheffield's East End.

Has anything really changed in Tinsley as a result? Health and local authorities jointly produced a Tinsley environment and health audit, and action plan (Sheffield City Council/Sheffield Health, 1999), with considerable input from the local community. Community research used focus groups and inter-views, health diaries, discussions at Tinsley Forum meetings and a large postal household survey. The plan which emerged identified six key areas for action: (1) traffic management and reduction; (2) noise reduction; (3) improving the physical environment; (4) better local facilities and services; (5) improving access and mobility in and around Tinsley; and (6) more local control and consideration of environment and health issues in future development plans. Community representatives have devoted many unpaid hours to the group's work yet progress, even on some relatively small environmental mitigation measures, such as noise attenuation or highways signage and regrading, has been painfully slow. The rhetoric of partnership has demanded much and, as yet, delivered little.

It is salutary to note that the most tangible outcome of the project's work in Tinsley, the Tinsley Tree project (a community enterprise with £0.3m of UK and European funding, providing employment and training for local people, and environmental improvement through tree planting) was achieved by the efforts of the community alone.

THE LOCAL AUTHORITY DILEMMA: RIDING TWO HORSES AT THE SAME TIME

The project brought into sharp focus the dilemma facing local authorities. They are charged with tackling social exclusion and reducing inequalities and also have a lead role to play in the economic development of the city and region. On one hand, they are falling over backwards to meet the demands of developers promising 'inward investment', jobs, economic revival (and threatening reloca-tion), and on the other seeking to work 'in partnership' with local communities on neighbourhood renewal and social inclusion.

Local communities' experience of the developer-led agenda, pursued relentlessly by the Sheffield Development Corporation in the 1980s and 1990s, has been one of exclusion from economic benefits and full exposure to social and environmental costs. Achieving sustainable regeneration requires a different approach to the mechanisms and purposes of economic development – 'being prepared to think in different ways and to find new ways to do things' (DETR, 1999b). However, recent research into sustainable development as a public policy issue found that, in practice, when it comes to inward investment, 'there remain competing policy objectives which have not been resolved and which the current institutional framework militates against resolving' (DETR, 2000c). The conclusion – that corporate economic objectives tend to dominate, so that unsus-tainable development continues – resonates with our experience in Sheffield. The local authority is in the uncomfortable position of being a schizophrenic ref-eree between local democracy, on the one hand, and corporate power, on the other.

WHAT COMES NEXT?

The East End Quality of Life initiative

In late 1999 the East End Quality of Life initiative (EEQOL) was established with health action zone funding, under the auspices of the East End Strategy Group, and is developing health impact assessment as a participatory tool to scrutinize transport, planning and development policies for this area of Sheffield. Compared with the Tinsley project, this initiative takes on a bigger area with at least 18,000 residents, more complex issues, and uneven community structures. It directly tackles the economic orthodoxy that the city's regeneration is best served, above all, by the need to secure inward investment and growth which, in turn, means meeting developers' demands for more roads and car parking space. This mindset, held by many local authority planners and elected members, is often justified by the claim that benefits will 'trickle down' to those most in need. Yet there is much compelling evidence to the contrary, from the East End itself and also from national and international studies of regeneration. The same mindset seems blind to the social and environmental costs of such a development strategy – widening health inequalities which impose an increasing burden on shrinking public services and inadequately supported community infrastructures.

The launch of EEQOL coincided with a major local authority study into the future development of the area around the M1 motorway, which includes Sheffield's East End and a number of development sites in Rotherham. The area under consideration is one of three 'strategic economic zones' designated within South Yorkshire's Objective One programme. The brief for the planning study included references to wide consultation, working closely with EEQOL on health impacts, and with local environmental protection services on environmental impacts. Yet in practice environmental, health and community considerations were all marginalized. A detailed prospective and participatory Health Impact Assessment (HIA) was not possible, as many of the assumptions and data underlying the report were not made public. The study proposed some radical public transport solutions, including a major extension to Sheffield's light rail system, and some references to green travel plans and tight car parking guidelines. But these were undermined by plans for highway enhancements, such as a new four-lane road to increase the capacity of M1 Junction 34S, where nitrogen dioxide levels are already 30 to 50 per cent over national air quality strategy objectives, and which lies in the centre of an air quality management area. The EEQOL HIA on the planning study makes a number of proposals designed to increase the health benefits and reduce the health damage of the proposed strategy (East End Quality of Life, 2000b). Time will tell what influence the HIA has on the final strategy adopted.

THE EAST END STANDING CONFERENCE

EEQOL was instrumental in the East End Strategy Group's establishment of a standing conference where developers, community and voluntary sector representatives come together, with the local authority as arbitrator, to debate the dilemmas in achieving sustainable local regeneration. The conference brings the community face to face with developers; will that lead to a better understanding of the community's aspirations? Debating these issues in such a forum may make it clear that the community perspective on regeneration includes not only job creation, but also job quality, local access to jobs, social and environmental impacts of development, quality and accessibility of public services, and community involvement in decision-making.

CONCLUSION

The Health For All focus on health inequalities, participation and inter-agency working taken by both the projects described here has the potential to be a powerful integrative and emancipatory force. But our experience also demonstrates strong forces opposing new ways of thinking and doing that sustainable development requires, which result in the marginalization of democracy and the suffocating embrace of corporate power in every aspect of our lives.

Where will the commitment and drive for change come from? Our experience suggests that joining forces with the local communities most marginalized and damaged by past economic development policies may be the most effective, perhaps the *only*, way of bringing about change. Alliances of health, regeneration and environmental interests can make an impact, but unless they ally with local communities and tackle head-on the mainstream economic agenda and the institutional framework that supports it, they will remain marginalized. Current UK government and EU policies contain many exhortations to invigorate local democracy and place communities at the centre of decision-making. In our attempts to turn this rhetoric into reality, we may find important allies within regional, national and international bodies. It is also vital to develop and strengthen the community infrastructure and build community capacity to participate in strategic development decisions. Local action is to some extent limited by larger global forces; yet resistance can be strengthened and focused by decisions and actions which clearly have no regard for the livelihoods of local people. We can learn much from community campaigns around the world, especially from the South, where there is long experience of action to safeguard livelihoods (and the environmental resources upon which these depend) from threats posed by global economic policies. In the words of Redclift (1984), 'perhaps we should take our cues from societies whose very existence "development" has always threatened'.

2.3

ENVIRONMENTAL JUSTICE

Eurig Scandrett

Environmentally mediated causes of ill health have particular features which make health promotion work in this area both important and challenging. The causes of ill health are often diffuse, complex, have multiple origins and are difficult to identify because of interactions with other factors. The environmental damage arises from the external effects of economic activity and the health impacts are socially concentrated. The common material interests of those groups mainly affected by environmentally mediated ill health provide an opportunity for collective action for structural change which can lead to social and political, as well as public health, improvements.

The value of sustainable development as a discourse acceptable to divergent interests has been noted (e.g. Jacobs, 1999). For example, a European model of ecological modernization has been proposed as a means of integrating environmental and business agendas to produce 'win-win' solutions (Blowers, 1997). Such market-led mechanisms, however, maintain the existing unequal distribution of environmental benefit and harm. In response, an alternative discourse of environmental justice is emerging from grassroots campaigns throughout the world, primarily around health-related environmental damage, providing a potential challenge to complacent sustainable development. Friends of the Earth Scotland sees itself as a campaign for environmental justice, in which the multiple demands of social, global and intergenerational equity must be addressed.

Guha and Martinez-Alier (1997) argue that there is a distinct materialist environmentalism, or 'environmentalism of the poor' in the poor countries of the South as well as among exploited groups in the capitalist West. The materialist environmentalists are concerned with the defence of natural resources and environments which are needed for their livelihood, and which are threatened by capital expansion or the state. While a more significant force among the poor in the poorer countries, they also identify materialist environmentalists in the affluent countries who react against the 'effluence of affluence' which threatens their own livelihood, health and well-being. Guha and Martinez-Alier's model is useful for the analysis of popular resistance to environmentally damaging activities in Western countries, of which the most politically significant is the environmental justice movement in the USA.

This network of some 5,000 black, Hispanic and indigenous grassroots communities has organized against the pollution effects of environmental racism – the preferential siting of environmentally hazardous facilities in black neighbourhoods and in indigenous peoples' reservations (e.g. Bullard, 1993; Capek, 1993; Stevens, 1998). North American racism has its roots in English colonialism and slave-owning, in which Scotland participated keenly; it has been argued that the 1707 Act of Union was motivated by Scotland's desire to share in England's colonial expansion (Hunter, 1994). However, the institutionalization of racism in the UK has taken different forms and environmental injustices appear to be determined primarily by class (although see Agyeman and Evans, 1996).

Stevens (1998) argues that the environmental justice movement emerged in the USA in the mid-1970s as a result of an acceleration in the process of capital globalization. This weakened both the power of the state to regulate, and of the labour movement to resist, creating the increasing economic and social fragmentation of peripheral communities. The onslaught led to the eruption of a social movement, riding on the back of the black civil rights movement of the 1960s.

The social and geographical concentration of the adverse external effects of capitalist development occurs both globally (Lewis, 1999) and locally (Boardman et al., 1999), and also around regional economic blocs. Scotland, as a peripheral European country, tends to be seen both as a source of primary natural resources and a sink for unwanted waste, with low regulation standards and practices (Scandrett et al., 2000).

The global economy of resource consumption can be analysed in different ways. Guha and Martinez-Alier (1997) calculate the ecological debt owed by rich countries to the South for their history of resource exploitation. Internationally, Friends of the Earth has used the concept of environmental space, based on an equal distribution of resource consumption per capita, within limits determined by extractable resource stock and the absorption capacity of the waste stream (Carley and Spapens, 1998; McLaren et al., 1998).

Friends of the Earth Scotland's conception of environmental justice therefore brings together the need for global and intergenerational equity in resource consumption and ecological and social health, with a priority to act with those who are the victims of inequality in the present. This is succinctly summarized in FoE Scotland's slogan 'no less than a decent environment for all, no more than our fair share of the Earth's resources'.

Some have argued for a rights-based approach to environmental justice and various opportunities for this exist. Though neither explicitly include an environmental right, both the European Convention on Human Rights as incorporated into Scots and English law (Thornton and Tromans, 1999), and the United Nations Declaration of Human Rights (Williams, 1998) can be interpreted as covering environmentally mediated human rights abuses. Hayward (2000) advocates a specific constitutional environmental right for Scotland and Friends of the Earth has lobbied for the inclusion of such a right in the Northern Ireland Bill of Rights. The constitution of South Africa includes the provision that 'every person shall have the right to an environment which is not detrimental to his or her health or well-being' (Article 29, Act 200, 1993).

A rights-based approach is beneficial but inadequate. Legal and constitutional rights are available equally to all individuals, who have access to redress through state or court procedures. But a social understanding of environmental justice recognizes existing inequality and asserts the possibility of a collective means of redress.

Even where rights exist, their application is patchy and favours powerful interests. Access to public data is often refused (FoES, 1992) and regulators have a poor record in reporting offenders (Matthews, 1994): for example, local authorities and the Scottish Environment Protection Agency (SEPA) make inadequate use of enforcement mechanisms (McBride, 1999), leading to poor identification of pollution and low referral rates to procurators fiscal. When prosecution is successful, court imposed fines are low (ENDS, 1998b, 1999).

Existing structures of accountability are inadequate. Land-use planning has a presumption in favour of development. Public participation is largely reactive with no right of appeal at present. Company law requires accountability only to investors, and both public bodies and private companies too often operate in a culture of secrecy. Polluting operations have virtually no accountability to their local community.

In such a climate, health promotion often means working for greater accountability in the economy, as the case studies below will demonstrate. Each arises from conflicts over waste management. As the final destination of all resources and the end of the line in economic externality, waste makes a useful index of environmental justice. The industry is worth £350m in Scotland (£4.1bn in Britain) and employs about 9,000 people (Biffa, 1997; SEPA, 1999). Although evidence is scant, waste management facilities are frequently sited near to communities with low social and economic status (G. Harbison, personal communication) and increased health problems have been reported in populations living near to landfills and incinerators (Dolk et al., 1998; Vrijheid et al., 1998). Moreover, the management of waste is a crucial challenge for sustainability. Scotland's national waste strategy aims for waste management earlier in the waste hierarchy, although we are starting from a poor position (SEPA, 1999).

GREENGAIRS

The North Lanarkshire community of Greengairs is surrounded by opencast coal mines and landfill sites. In 1998, soil contaminated with polychlorinated biphenyls (PCBs) was imported from Hertfordshire by waste company Shanks & McEwan to one of their landfills in Greengairs (ENDS, 1998a). Although the level of PCB contamination was higher than that permitted for deposition in any landfill in England or Wales, the licence for the Greengairs site permitted higher levels of contamination.

The community mobilized to resist this toxic import. By blockading the site the community forced concessions from Shanks & McEwan, including an end to the toxic dumping and economic benefits for the community.

The factors leading to this example are illustrative. In local structure plans, devastated areas are favoured for the development of landfill, which leads to a concentration of environmentally damaging activity around particular communities. Negligence on the part of SEPA led to a failure to upgrade Shanks & McEwan's licence at Greengairs, and the company was fast to exploit this loophole. The action of the community forced a more direct local account-ability than was achieved either by planning or operational regulations.

DOUGLAS

In Dundee, after years of protest from the local community of Douglas sup-ported by FoE Scotland, a waste incinerator was finally closed in 1996 when European emission regulations were tightened up. Plans for an improved 'waste to energy' incinerator were opposed by both the community and FoE, but per-mission was nonetheless granted and the plant was built in 1999 under a public–private partnership company, Dundee Energy Recycling Limited (DERL). Despite opposing incineration as a means of waste management, FoE worked with the community to explore how the company could be made more accountable. Agreement was reached between the community and the com-pany to negotiate a 'good neighbour agreement'.

Good neighbour agreements have been used in the USA to provide a degree of accountability by large industries to their neighbouring communities. The DERL / Douglas agreement, the first in the UK, commits the company to regular negotiations with community representatives; providing accessible information; consulting on emergency planning; improving environmental per-formance; ensuring sensitive lorry routes and times; and encouraging local employment and economic development. While they do not amount to full local economic democracy, good neighbour agreements do provide some industry accountability to significant stakeholders (Lewis and Henkels, 1998).

KAIMES

Kirknewton, a small community on the western boundary of Edinburgh, is overlooked by Kaimes hill from which basalt was quarried for ten years from 1977. Following extraction, Kings & Company, who operated the site, sought to restore it by depositing waste material in the void left by the quarry working. Consent was given for this, although the community assumed that the quarry would be quickly restored after the end of its working life. Yet only days before the expiry of their own deadline to restore the site, the city council awarded a ten-year contract to the waste disposal company now operating the site to take millions of tons of the city's rubbish to the site.

Neither planning permission for the continued operation of the site, nor technical details of the site restoration, could be produced by the city council. Legal opinion was sought by the local community, which confirmed not only that the site lacked appropriate planning permission, but also that the original decision by the council to permit waste dumping for site rehabilitation had been illegal.

The council repeatedly failed to respond to requests for information, and awarded a further contract to the company after assurances were given by coun-cil officials that there were no outstanding planning issues to be resolved. The group initiated judicial review in the Court of Session but at the eleventh hour, the council (which acts both as the planning and the waste disposal authority) conceded that it was at fault, and started enforcement action against the current operators, Hanson Waste Management.

These case studies demonstrate how communities can challenge environmental injustices by wresting some accountability from economic power, by demanding existing rights (Kaimes), by negotiating additional concessions (Douglas) and by exerting power through direct action (Greengairs). These tactics mirror those of the labour movement in which defence of workers' health through economic democracy has involved implementing health and safety legislation, through locally negotiated improvements and through industrial militancy.

Using an environmental justice approach opens up new possibilities for grassroots alliances between environmentalists and community or trade union activists, and is being widely pursued (Permanent People's Tribunal on Industrial Hazards and Human Rights, 1998). The ideas of environmental justice are being developed from below, by those who directly suffer the 'side effects' of economic activity.

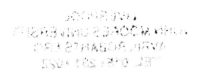

3

COMMUNITY DEVELOPMENT

Mary Amos

This chapter provides a theoretical and historical overview of community development (CD) and health, and explores its relationship with practice in public health and health promotion. It highlights the struggles to increase social capital, strengthen public participation and bring about increased opportunities for health improvement, especially by those most marginalized, and identifies underlying issues in theory and evaluation, before going on to look at the future of CD as a tool for health. The purpose is to share practice and deepen understanding and acceptance of CD as central to improving health.

DEFINITIONS AND DEVELOPMENTS

Since the 1970s, the changing fortunes of CD in health promotion have tended to vary along with the tensions between theory and practice. Since CD is a political activity based on collective experience and action, it has remained at odds with the focus on personal behaviour which has dominated mainstream policy and practice. An examination of CD for health is therefore of pivotal importance to any study of health promotion. We will consider the radical traditions of CD based on a socialist ideology of fighting injustices which impact upon the health of some more than others and 'the current neo-liberal approach to citizenship which places obligations above rights and in which capitalism (unregulated free-market global expansion) destroys communities and social institutions' (Jordan, 1998).

There are some important definitions to be set out before examining CD for health. In 1948, the United Nations' definition of CD linked an emerging idea of community empowerment to modern concerns with community organizing and power. The UN definition of CD was 'a movement to promote better living for the whole community, with active participation and if possible on the initiative of the community, but if this initiative is not forthcoming, by the use of techniques for arousing it and stimulating it' (Craig, 1989). The Standing Conference on Community Development published its own definition of CD as a charter (1995), from which two statements help to clarify CD as a process: 'Community development is crucially concerned with the issues of powerlessness and disadvantage: as such it should involve all members of society, and offers a practice that is part of social change'; 'Community development is about the active involvement of people sharing in the issues which affect their lives. It is a process based on the sharing of power, skills, knowledge and experience.' CD is radical in intent – it aims to challenge the status quo and force changes which move power in favour of the powerless.

CD for health is inextricably linked with consciousness-raising and change, and has its contemporary origins in the political movements of the 1960s and in developing countries where colonial oppression held back human rights. Earlier forms of 'community development' in Victorian England adopted a paternalistic approach to improving the lot of the poor, which was replicated in British outposts, particularly in West Africa, before World War II by the Colonial Office in the form of self-help projects. During the post-war period CD programmes in 'Third World' countries were designed to pave the way for the transition to independence, but the approach of international agencies was 'top down' and 'giving power' with the intention that a country move towards a western, capitalist model of government. Training for CD workers was still very much *for* people and not *with* people. Other countries, such as China, Cuba and Tanzania searched for alternative solutions to conventional health development and developed socialist strategies. WHO, in its report *Health by the People* (1975), noted that 'these countries had a clear advantage in starting primary health care change if they came from such a starting point politically'.

CD is therefore both a philosophy and a way of working, which are mutually supporting – the action–reflection–action loop. The philosophy of CD for health recognizes the injustice of inequalities in society which manifest themselves as poor health and early death and sees political action on a broad front as essential. Like most ways of working for change, CD for health is radical in intent and outcome but may encounter repressive tolerance – a false acceptance in order to block change. The distinctive contribution of the CD approach to community health work is that the focus is on reducing people's sense of powerlessness and on increasing equity and access which challenges medical power. Such work is concerned with developing power relations between groups and institutions.

Working with communities to encourage informed and powerful partnerships is a key function of CD. This could be the role of any statutory agency as well as the voluntary sector and has its roots in social movements such as feminism, anti-racism or the self-help movement. During the 1980s a 'community development and health' movement developed with a wide base of supporters exchanging ideas and initiating work, much of it outside mainstream NHS funding. Community health projects used empowerment, advocacy and support – both personal and collective – in their work with communities. Smithies and Webster (1998) chart the development of the national profile of CD and health work during the 1970s and 1980s which brought together projects, groups and radical professionals. They comment: 'The Labour government, elected in May 1997, has wasted little time in bringing forward policies to reform and develop the NHS and work to promote the health of the UK population . . . it remains to be seen how many of these will impact community involvement in practice.' They also provide case studies which demonstrate good practice using different techniques that operate at various levels such as inter-agency or inter-community working. Organizational development is highlighted as a key element in the

community participation process, since once communities are used to participation, then it follows that organizations require skills, knowledge and systems
to enable them to work collaboratively. There is a general 'slipperiness' in the literature, with 'community development' and 'community participation' used
almost interchangeably. One distinction may be the intention: is participation
designed to 'allow' decision-making in statutory agency-led agendas or in community-led agendas? The former might be called 'capacity-building for social
control' while the latter is 'capacity-building for social change'.

Community participation, or more accurately 'communities participation'
is a vital element in the communities development model, but clearly there are
different applications according to intention – to transform power bases or to
take part in decision-making. This is not to devalue community involvement in
decision-making, an essential part of democratic systems. Governance, the
process of collectively sorting out problems to meet society's needs, is emerging
in local government approaches to city health plans and is strongly influenced
by WHO's healthy cities movement. Building on the principles set out in the
1978 Alma Ata declaration, the healthy cities movement was based on the
insights that the 'promotion of health must include the adaptation and transformation of those social structures that foster ill health, and that community
participation is the most powerful method of attaining this goal . . . backed up by
the development of appropriate health policies at both local and national levels'
(Campbell et al., 1999).

Community participation is a mantra in many national and international
documents – the Health For All by the Year 2000 strategy (WHO, 1981), the
Ottawa Charter for Health Promotion (WHO, 1986) which cites 'strengthening communities' as one of the necessary levels of action required to reduce inequalities
in health; the *Sundsvall Statement on Supportive Environments for Health* (WHO,
1991b), *Our Healthier Nation* (Department of Health, 1998). Indeed, a King's
Fund report examining the neighbourhood as a setting for health in relation to
a multitude of recent government initiatives (SureStart, New Deal for
Communities, Local Agenda 21, Healthy Living Centres, Supporting Families –
all of which emphasize local people's participation), warns:

> Neighbourhoods are likely to need support from a variety of resources to
> develop and sustain progress . . . The appointment of development and sup-
> port workers to work with local people . . . could greatly aid this process . . .
> The role does not require the creation of a new profession, nor should it nec-
> essarily signal a return to the 1970s model of community development.
> (Gowman, 1999)

The report does not elaborate on the '1970s model', but implies that CD may
have to reinvent itself to 'capacity build' for health and become acceptable to
current thinking.

The phrase 'capacity building' has come to mean building support, skills,
confidence and trust within communities, to become agents for their own health.
Skinner (1997) defines capacity building as:

> Development work that strengthens the ability of community organisations
> and groups to build their structures, systems, people and skills so that they

are better able to define and achieve their objectives and engage in consultation and planning, manage community projects and take part in partnerships and community enterprises. It includes aspects of training, organisational and personal development and resource building, organised in a planned and self-conscious manner, reflecting the principles of empowerment and equality.

As 'agents for health', one role for communities would be to work within existing structures to improve health where possible. As Grossman and Scala (1993) point out, there is no particular system for health as there is for education, sport or health care. Changes to systems within organizations have to be introduced in ways which make sense to the organization. But in the wider-ranging approach advocated by CD, communities act as 'agents for change for health' – a role which involves challenging structures which negate health. Health promotion is a challenging organizational task, so it is not surprising that infrastructures for health promotion are extremely underdeveloped.

Change at senior level, with grass-roots support, is vital to promoting public health: for example, activities such as an intergenerational event in a local community centre need to be resourced by an enlightened management which argues for outcomes such as breaking down fear and prejudice to be viewed as health outcomes. Jordan (1998) observes that there are tensions between free-market individualism and democratic collective responsibility and notes:

> The communitarian turn of the 1980s has shifted attention towards the virtues of active democratic citizenship, and the qualities of a sustainable culture of collective responsibility. But it is one thing to prescribe participation in the common good through inclusive democratic practices, and quite another to develop a policy programme for the reintegration of the poor, the regeneration of community spirit or the reinvention of civil society.

Aspects of community participation can be seen in contemporary discussions of public health (Jewkes and Murcott, 1996), but the notion of a *duty* to participate is anathema to CD practice, as is participation in order to consolidate the power of the bureaucracy. Labonte (1999) reminds us that, 'The health of people of the planet ultimately requires a new global regulatory framework. But even as efforts to this end are undertaken, there is a need to develop new local coping strategies. Many of these already are the hallmarks of community development.' The relationship between community participation and CD is close and holds the potential to redistribute power if the intentions of the work, at whatever level, are made explicit. This requires a sound understanding of the theories behind such work.

THEORETICAL ROOTS OF COMMUNITY DEVELOPMENT

The theoretical basis for CD and health lies in three main areas: social organization, power and control, and lay perspectives of health. These link up with theories of personal and community empowerment and together have informed the thinking and practice of CD workers and strategists. Paulo Freire, the Brazilian educationalist and philosopher, developed a theory of empowering education in his work with communities: that education was concerned with human liberation and that all participants in the process were equals and co-learners; learners might uncover the root causes of their place in society by critical dialogue (Freire, 1973). This goes beyond understanding and leads to action to rectify the situation. Two major perspectives have been used to explain social change: functionalist and conflict views. Functionalists see social change as a gradual, adaptive process orientated towards system reform based on co-operation. Social change theories based on the conflict view see change as occurring when one of several interests in a system gains ascendancy. Those who control important parts of the system, particularly the economic and political sectors, establish the social norms.

CD for health attempts, as part of wider political action, to shift the influence in favour of communities who do not have power and control and who suffer the worst health. The two system-level theories provide a framework for describing macro systems, but it is the process theories about community change that have most influenced health promotion. These include theories at the individual, organizational, community and environmental levels. Individual-level theories of change have influenced the mainstream of health promotion activity, based on techniques of influencing personal decisions about health such as the Health Belief Model, the Theory of Reasoned Action, Social Learning Theory and the Trans-theoretical Model (Naidoo and Wills, 2001). Of course, the limitations of personal or lifestyle health promotion activities have been well documented (Adams and Pintus 1994; Benzeval et al., 1995; McQueen, 1989; Whitehead, 1987).

Strategies that include multi-level approaches to health promotion, with CD acting as a bridge between one level and another, have been advocated. But simply setting two different models alongside one another may remain problematic (Whitelaw et al., 1997). The models come from conflicting paradigms – the individual bio-medical approach and the political–social action approach. Creating a framework which tries to create an all-embracing picture in which equal weight is given to each component may be offering an image of progressiveness while changing nothing. The risk is that this allows traditional practice (personal behaviour change) to simply continue under the guise of a more radical approach. Health promotion practice in Britain has to a great extent focused on personal behaviour, albeit sometimes in community settings. There have been exceptions to this in several areas of the country, but often 'community' health promotion has been little more than personal health promotion activity carried out with groups in community settings, for example, safer sex education in a youth club or stress management in a workplace. But the radical traditions on which CD for health is based aim to create alliances for campaigning and advocacy on the fundamental determinants of health inequalities.

Theoretical approaches for change at community level have been formulated. Rothman (1979, 1996) describes three general ways to intervene in a community to achieve change: locality development, social planning and social action. Locality development emphasizes the participation of local residents in identifying and solving problems, often with the help of a change agent. The social planning approach is based on rational planning and problem-solving involving communities as consumers of the process rather than equal partners. By contrast, the social action approach is usually based on conflict and requires a dramatic shift in power, usually in favour of disadvantaged groups. Clearly the radical roots of CD are in the social action approach and locality development. A number of recent studies suggest that community members take on aspects of capacity building (Jackson et al., 1994), community development (Labonte, 1993) and community 'regeneration' (McKnight, 1987), all of which are orientated to returning more power and control to the community.

Rissel (1994) helps to make an important distinction about the central construct of health promotion – that of empowerment. The distinction between psychological empowerment (the subjective feeling of feeling greater control) and community empowerment (the objective reality of greater power following a reallocation of resources) is often blurred in CD work for health. While it is reasonable to suggest that one follows the other – the personal leading to the collective – this may not always or often be the case. By enhancing participation in collective action, a raised sense of community contributes to the likelihood that the community is empowered. It might be expected that groups with actual control over resources have a high level of reported psychological empowerment, although the reverse is not true (Bracht, 1999). The concept of a continuum of community empowerment has been developed by several authors (Bracht, 1999) illustrating the process of personal development followed by mutual development and coalitions for social action. The process may not be a linear one moving from one stage to another. For example, joining a mutual support group may lead first to personal empowerment; in addition, individuals may or may not choose to participate in social actions.

EVALUATION

Theoretical principles inform the methodology and evaluation of CD work for health. Concepts of health held by different sections of society – lay concepts – form the basis for any CD for health work. Cornwell (1984) described how private and public accounts of health differ: the former being more holistic and social. Blaxter (1990) identified gender and class differences in explanations of health and ill health. Oakley et al. (1992) used qualitative research to highlight socially structured discrimination by gender and ethnicity in relation to smoking. Jones (undated) documented ten years of achievements of the Pilton Health Project which challenges medical dominance over health. Social science's perspective on health being socially and economically constructed provides a critique of scientific medicine. The dominant evidence-based medical paradigm is resistant to the new and emerging holistic interpretations of health upon which inter-agency and inter-community strategies are built. There are particular difficulties when agreeing how success should be judged or measured, and of course conflict between the biomedical approach to evaluation and CD is not new (Allison and Rootman, 1996; Beattie, 1995; Bjaras et al., 1991; Hepworth, 1997). According to Beattie, these different approaches to evaluation have become polarized into 'two warring camps' – one drawing on the traditions of quantitative evaluation in terms of managerial audit (economy, efficiency and effectiveness, sometimes with equity added) and the other focusing on people, places and processes drawn from disciplines such as education, community work and health in developing countries.

More recently the relevance of social approaches to the organization and delivery of public health has received attention at a national level (Campbell et al., 1999). The Health Education Authority investigated the idea of social capital and set out to establish empirical links between aspects of social capital and health outcomes. It concluded that social capital has the potential 'to make a valuable contribution to . . . what constitutes a "health enabling" community'. However, one danger of not acknowledging the philosophical, ideological and practical differences between community *development* work for health and community-*based* work for health is that collaboration between agencies or communities becomes a pretence, and so the struggles for social equity are weakened. Stevenson and Burke (1991) tellingly note that 'with its emphasis on an organic harmony and consensus among diverse identities and its tendency to develop methodological "resolutions" to political problems, health promotion mystifies rather than clarifies the nature of social barriers to meaningful change'. Pluralistic evaluation, which presents a range of different kinds of information from different sources, is required in the multi-sector and multi-level work for health that is flowing from current public policy initiatives such as Health Action Zones, Health Improvement Programmes and the like. Community participation methods have been successfully applied to health-related interventions and measured using process indicators (Bjaras et al., 1991). Hepworth (1997) locates CD within her health outcome differentiation types, placing it as a social health outcome. In this expansion of 'health' outcomes, changes in the 'enhancers of health' can be evaluated as structural, social and community conditions as well as biomedical health outcomes. Improvements in these conditions for health are important measures, which only become problematic when they are compared within a biomedical paradigm.

Barr et al., (1996) developed a comprehensive series of core indicators flexible enough to apply to a range of settings and scales of operation. The indicators are presented as ten building blocks concerned with community empowerment and community quality of life. Such work could provide a valuable planning and evaluation framework for intersectoral health promotion strategies with CD at their centre, and help to monitor performance in terms of the match between community aspirations and what agencies actually do. CD as a tool to promote health is part of a political movement and so it seems inappropriate to 'evaluate' it as if it were a technical and precise intervention. Petersen (1996) argues that while limited reforms have been achieved through community participation in public health, there has been a failure to go beyond local concerns to nurture a movement for broader change. Ife (1995) points out that participation may be little more than tokenism as people often have very limited power to really influence decisions, and may end up co-opted into a structure that they originally set out to oppose. The evaluation of processes and outcomes of CD for health sit within theories of change – personal, organizational and community – and should be as open to critical appraisal as any other; proponents and critics alike would agree that it is not acceptable to work in this way just because it is 'inherently good' to do so. Health Action Zones are using theories of change and realistic evaluation to systematically and cumulatively evaluate complex community initiatives (Judge, 2000).

Poland (1996), in considering the healthy cities movement, suggests that what is needed is a 'critical pedagogy' which would engage participants in reflexive examination of the nature of social organization and the root causes of health, coupled with an awareness of community organizing strategies, with which to develop a progressive social change agenda, and as a context for healthy public policy development at a local level. The critical learning experience extolled here is a challenge for all participants in CD and health work. Labonte (1999) argues that health promotion will be challenged to act on the two fronts that underpinned health promotion a century ago: social justice (reducing inequalities in wealth and power) and healthy environments (increasing sustainable social and economic practices), which will 'require a shift in the ideology of many health promotion employers from one of content (dissemination of health knowledge to reduce individual risk factors) to one of context (changing social relations of power to reduce economically structured risk conditions)'.

THE FUTURE OF CD FOR HEALTH

The idea of 'evidence-based health promotion' (WHO, 1999b) creates new challenges for health promoters, but should certainly include CD as a tool to achieve the goals of the healthy cities programme. To enable the matrices of partnerships across groupings to be mutually empowering, challenges and constraints must be faced. Mayo (1997) summarizes the positive features of such partnerships as providing extra resources, tackling paternalism, developing reciprocity (mutually beneficial exchange) and social solidarity (connectedness and concern for others). But there are negatives too – those inherent in the wider policy framework and those that relate to implementation. Examples might help here: the policy framework for partnerships in community regeneration frequently contains proposals to further deregulate the planning system and encourage a growth in markets, with outcomes measured in 'flagship' private property development rather than local, social regeneration. Urban regeneration and CD are further impacted upon negatively at implementation level by such practices as the competitive nature of bidding for funds against other proposals, which does not assist the sustainability of local area initiatives. Other market-led approaches such as short-term funding, on the premise that exit strategies have to be developed to sustain the work once funding is withdrawn, have divided rather than united partners. The 'neighbourhood', together with schools and workplaces, is cited as a vital partner in a 'contract for health' in the government's White Paper *Our Healthier Nation* (Department of Health, 1998), but support and development of community action to achieve this are less evident. Current evidence (Duncan and Thomas, 2000) suggests that, in neighbourhood renewal strategies, CD work is not a priority for many programmes and is still vulnerable to cuts; indeed, there is some indication that the number of CD workers has declined.

There are inherent tensions between statutory organizations and CD for health which challenge the processes and actions of those organizations. How can unequal power bases such as neighbourhood projects or minority groups compete without support and how can CD workers represent the interests of different communities at the same time? Conflict is inevitable. While paid and unpaid community developers engage in time- and energy-consuming exercises such as writing funding bids or making links, the communities they seek to engage may be cynical due to over-consultation, apparent lack of progress or simple pessimism. Are the 'values' held within CD work – social justice, fairness, concern for community, neighbourliness, cohesion, acceptance of others – still possible given the void left by the 1980s' economic and social depletion? There is an issue here about the willingness and ability of communities to work together for collective health gain. In turn, the ability of CD to build infrastructures for health promotion is open for debate. Who should be funding this work? How should it be sustained? Where does the strength of conceptual thinking come from?

Alternative forms of CD for health were suggested by Mayo (1997) based on the Association of Metropolitan Authorities' 'good practice' guidelines, which recognized that CD strategies should reflect the need for communities' independent support and expertise. However effectively they are supported from the public sector, managers and workers as well as elected representatives need adequate training to see the process as a positive challenge rather than a threat. CD cannot deal with big issues such as poverty and the marginalization of many groups in society. If supported by public policies that improve health equitably and by social movements such as ethical investing, social regeneration, anti-institutional racism, and so on, CD as a tool for health can be nourished. CD alone cannot change the structures of society but it can help people to feel more in control and can encourage activism. If health improvement strategies can be developed which address both structural barriers as well as building social and organizational capacity, then progress towards eradicating inequity in health may be made. Rather than swallow the idea that CD can be both radical and transforming while at the same time remain non-political and unchallenging to the status quo, policy-makers should support radical CD programmes which demand redistributive fiscal policy, the rebuilding of communities, and anti-exclusionary social policies.

ACKNOWLEDGEMENT

With thanks to Healthy Portsmouth at Portsmouth City Council, for allowing time to devote to this work.

3.1

THEORY, OPPORTUNITY, SERENDIPITY: COMMUNITY DEVELOPMENT IN SHEFFIELD

Martine Standish

Community development work has been around for many years. Community development and health work, however, is a rather newer animal, and given the uneasy relationship between 'pure' community development and the use of community development approaches to deliver centrally determined agendas, that animal has often seemed too much like a camel (that is, a horse designed by a committee). A real challenge for community development and health projects has too frequently been the reluctance of the committee, having released its camel, to welcome it back. In other words, agencies have established community development projects but failed to learn from them, or to make the organizational changes suggested by communities.

But things have improved. Over the past ten years or so clearer links have been made between community development, health promotion, organizational development and the 'health establishment', which have had real benefits for local people. In this case study I will try to illustrate this through a personal view of community development and health in Sheffield during these years. In particular, I will draw on the experience of working with the Healthy Sheffield Development Unit, the Heart of Our City community development and heart health project, the health promotion department's poverty team and, most recently, area action.

In 1988, I was co-ordinator of a women's health bus in Sheffield, providing screening and information. I certainly do not think many people regarded me then as a necessary element of mainstream provision. I saw myself as a unique and radical link between marginalized communities and the health service, and did not hope to influence the mainstream much. It was only as the approach to health promotion in the city changed (see Adams and Cunning, Chapter 1.3, this volume) that I recognized what I was doing as health promotion. Perhaps I was just a sadly isolated activist, but it seems more likely that the links between community development and the health services were far less clear then.

Healthy Sheffield made these links explicit. Community participation – supporting communities to participate meaningfully in the life of their city and to influence those things affecting their health – was a central approach of the Healthy Sheffield Partnership, and community development was seen as the way to bring about participation.

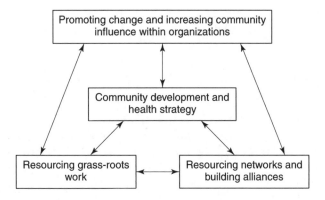

Figure 3.1.1 The three elements of a community development and health strategy

By 1993, Healthy Sheffield had reviewed existing community health projects and devised a strategy to support community development. This hinged on a model developed by the UK Health For All Network (1991) and shown in Figure 3.1.1.

It was clear that effective community development required all three key elements: resources for grass-roots work, support for networks and alliances, and organizational development. In retrospect, at that time we were better informed about how to support the first two elements; organizational develop-ment, though essential, was not yet tangible.

The Heart of Our City was a demonstration project for Healthy Sheffield, intended to show all three elements in action. It was launched in 1990 as an inno-vative six-year community development and heart health project, based in four inner-city wards. The first three years of funding came from the then Health Education Authority heart health programme, inevitably creating a tension between central polices and local interests: national funding was available for projects on heart health, but the community development approach meant find-ing out what local people were concerned about and wanted to act on. The project also attempted to reconcile and act on differing analyses of the causes of heart disease – one based on an individual behaviour focus (smoking, diet and exercise as set out in *Health of the Nation*, Department of Health, 1992), the other concerned with the socioeconomic and psychosocial roots of heart disease (Hunt, 1994; Williams and Popay, 1994). The national agenda, and therefore project funding, became increasingly dominated by the individual risk factor approach during the life of the project.

Heart of Our City aimed to promote heart health through a range of inter-ventions, some of which are shown in Box 3.1.1. The project also applied community development approaches to its evaluation, recruiting and training local community researchers who also helped disseminate findings (Standish, 1995). This was a big agenda for a small team – at its largest, the project employed a co-ordinator, two community development workers, a primary health care development worker, an information officer and a researcher for a target population of 65,000. After the first three years, the team was reduced.

BOX 3.1.1   HEART OF OUR CITY: SOME APPROACHES
USED

- Building skills, confidence and knowledge in individuals, through the provision of information, training and involvement in project activities.
- Initiating and supporting local self-help and community groups (e.g. a group for those in the 40–60 age group).
- Bringing community groups and agencies together into local networks (e.g. an Environment and Health Forum in the Firth Park ward).
- Promoting activities around individual risk factors (e.g. healthy eating sessions and smoking cessation).
- Providing support to specifically targeted communities (e.g. Yemeni Men's Exercise Group).
- Sponsoring and supporting initiatives to improve local circumstances (e.g. anti-racism campaign, improvements to local parks and open spaces, community allotments).
- Working with health professionals to improve detection and treatment of heart disease (e.g. primary health care teams, community-based rehabilitation programmes).
- Engaging local businesses in heart health, particularly in promoting healthy eating.

The final evaluation of the project, jointly carried out by the two Sheffield universities, found impressive levels of awareness of the project and, to a lesser degree, involvement in its activities, alongside some positive changes in health-related beliefs and awareness of the causes of coronary heart disease. (It also noted that heart disease was not a high health priority for the community, emphasizing the tension between central policies and local interests.) In terms of individual risk factors, there were some behaviour changes – reductions in smoking, an increase in physical activity and dietary change – which suggested that the 'cost per life-year gained' of the project could be very low. On a broader community development assessment, the project had succeeded in stimulating local networks and building alliances, as well as helping a small number of local residents gain marketable skills or leadership qualities.

The project had been intended, throughout its life and beyond, to influence the activities of Healthy Sheffield partner agencies by bringing community needs to their attention. The final evaluation could only briefly consider those policy changes achieved during the lifetime of the project, such as the provision of women-only swimming sessions by the council to encourage Muslim women to make use of facilities. Some areas proved far more resistant to change: while some good work was done with local shops on promoting healthy eating, overall, the project was unable to effectively engage the local business community.

The Heart of Our City exit strategy was developed with a local steering group of residents and workers. The residents were very clear that the single most important element to retain was some community development worker time. The health authority was persuaded to continue to provide extra support in two areas with particular needs. In one, Burngreave, a community development and health worker was funded by the local community health care services, who would carry out grass-roots community development in a multicultural community, but also would encourage and support others with a community development role. In the second area, Parsons Cross, the health authority maintained a low level of funding to a voluntary community health project, which in turn preserved a community infrastructure in an area with few groups or resources. This continuity of community development input paid dividends when opportunities arose to attract new resources via a variety of government initiatives.

Other local policy initiatives have been at least partly attributable to the lessons learnt from Heart of Our City. The project highlighted the difficulty in bringing about individual behaviour change in the face of strong socio-economic obstacles: a stark example was the closure of a local shop that had supported the healthy eating campaign. As workers, our impression was that in six years the overall economic climate of the area deteriorated.

Our response was to establish a poverty team within the health promotion directorate to stimulate the health authority to consider what it could do locally to tackle poverty. We were assisted in developing our approach to poverty by Margaret Whitehead's analysis of the four levels of policy intervention to tackle inequalities: strengthening individuals; strengthening communities; improving access to essential facilities and services; and encouraging macro-economic and cultural change (Whitehead, 1995). Whitehead noted that most efforts had been directed at the first two levels. This helped us reflect on the work we had undertaken in the past, and identify gaps. For example, in Heart of Our City there was clearly little support from the macro-economic and cultural level for changes which would have encouraged individual and community development. As a checklist for ensuring that future initiatives addressed all four levels simultaneously, this proved an invaluable tool. Locally, we also developed a five-level model (Adams and Cunning, Chapter 1.3, this volume).

The health authority determined to work closely with the city council in four areas of the city with particularly poor health and severe deprivation. Two of these – Burngreave and Parsons Cross – had been within the Heart of Our City patch. Four health promotion specialists worked alongside local authority area co-ordinators and local communities, not to do grass-roots community development but to support the development of local infrastructures and engage the health service in addressing the needs of the communities. Their remit was to attract external resources into the area; strengthen community networks and structures so they could make use of resources to help themselves; help statutory agencies to respond more effectively to local needs; and make achievement of national health targets possible at a local level.

There is no blueprint for the support that the area action officers have provided. However, it is possible to identify a number of stages that are usually present when support for community development is initiated, including:

- mapping local stakeholders, including relevant citywide organizations, neighbourhood forums, community groups, local statutory services;
- needs assessment, involving members of the community;
- strategy development, working with the community to set short- and long-term objectives;
- working with the community to obtain resources, for example, regeneration funds, Health Action Zone funding;
- project and service development, obtaining resources for the community that address priorities such as childcare provision;
- organizational change, encouraging mainstream service providers to modify their operations to reflect the demands of the community, such as advocacy services within primary care.

To date, the area action initiative has proved very successful (see Box 3.1.2) in the priority areas, with activities reflecting the first three of Whitehead's levels. This work provided the basis for Sheffield's Health Action Zone bid, which attracted further resources to the four priority areas, and also influenced the use of major regeneration resources such as the Single Regeneration Budget (SRB) bids for the city, ensuring a health element. The third SRB round, in the Manor Castle area, was the first in the country to include health as an equal and integral part of the social and economic development plan. In the most recent round, which includes Parsons Cross, the health and social care strand includes funding of around £4m (out of a total £20m) for the seven-year programme. Similarly, in Burngreave, health is one of four strands in a New Deal for Communities initiative which is likely to bring £50m into that area over ten years. The co-ordinated area action approach has also allowed these different funding streams to be drawn together (with European funds in some cases) to support health promoting initiatives.

We are still building local capacity to support community development health work. The Community Health Educators' programme is one example of how we have drawn together work on poverty (and job creation), health information and access to health services, making use of regeneration funding. The

BOX 3.1.2   SOME SUCCESSES OF SHEFFIELD'S AREA ACTION INITIATIVE

- Developing the skills and confidence of individual community members, for example through the Community Health Educators' programme.
- Supporting projects to train local people to research the needs of their community.
- Developing the strength of local inter-agency and voluntary groups and their ability to manage projects and workers.
- Developing community forums that can attract resources and employ local people.
- Linking community participation to strategic planning.
- Encouraging services to respond to communities.

programme is co-ordinated on a citywide basis but delivered at an area level, and results in a pool of individuals from different communities with basic community development and health skills. The introduction to community development and health skills is an accredited course, with additional modules on information, advocacy, community research and training the trainers, and others to be developed. The Community Health Educators work with communities, in both unpaid and paid capacities, on health issues identified by the communities as important. They play a vital role in informing their communities about health issues, and in helping services to be more responsive to local needs. In one area, community health educators are already employed alongside primary health care staff to help develop specific services. In the future, we may see them establishing community enterprises to provide services. An adapted version of the course has also been developed for professional primary care staff.

So it does now seem that we have found some ways to make the crucial connections between community and organizational development. We still have to manage the tension between central priorities and local interests, but we have more scope to genuinely involve local people in setting local targets and deciding on methods of intervention. We also have some opportunities, via Health Action Zones, New Deal for Communities and other initiatives, to pilot interventions which may be taken up and lead to real changes at Whitehead's fourth level of macro-economic and cultural change.

Community development is increasingly recognized as an essential element of strategies to address health inequalities, but as the NHS goes through further changes there is a need to ensure that the capacity to support this is sustained. How can we support and utilize community development in the new NHS? Sheffield Health's area action officers currently have a role in both community development and organizational development. They are equipped with resources, skills and a value base to undertake development work in the community. They also function as managers within statutory organizations, with the status to link development work to agency development, and to provide support for other (more grass-roots) development workers.

The new primary care organizations emerging within the NHS will need the capacity to help community forums develop as functioning groups, able to plan effectively and employ staff, to support them to develop strategies to improve health and quality of life, and help them to respond effectively to community needs and proposals. In addition, they will need to provide management support to those undertaking development work, employ fresh skills as an organization, making use of local people as advocates, information workers or researchers, and assist mainstream workers to employ community development techniques.

It is important that community development is not used simply to help deliver particular, pre-determined, health programmes. Healthy Sheffield's community development strategy recommended ensuring that new and specialist services should not be funded at the expense of generic community development. A generic, sustained strategy of community development can develop workers with the skills and experience to build community infrastructures where there are none, and reveal as yet undiscovered health needs.

Looking back over work in community development and health in

Sheffield in the 1990s, I am struck first by what an incremental process it has been, each stage building on what has gone before. Community development is an open-ended commitment: you can set the direction you want to move in, but you do not always know exactly where you'll end up. Gazing back down the path travelled, however, it all makes sense. It is this tension between a planned approach, rooted in theory, and the necessary elements of opportunity and serendipity that make this a fascinating area of work. My second reflection is that we really have made progress over these years, especially in helping community development have an impact on statutory organizations and systems.

In Sheffield, we are still developing our use of community development approaches, finding new ways to apply them, new ways to support them and new ways to explain them to others. The clearer we have become about the principles which guide us, and the theories which support us, the more successful we have been. As we try to project ourselves into the new world beyond the next round of NHS changes, we need to remember to look back and see how we arrived here. Community development has been notoriously poorly recorded and remains little understood by policy-makers and NHS managers. It is worth tracing the steps and celebrating the progress.

ACKNOWLEDGEMENTS

With thanks to all my Sheffield colleagues, particularly Frances Cunning, Debbie Matthews, Gary McCulloch, Owen McDowell and Sue Greig.

3.2

USER MOVEMENTS, COMMUNITY DEVELOPMENT AND HEALTH PROMOTION

Marian Barnes

CONTESTED COMMUNITIES

Community has been a focus for sociological research and analysis for many years (see, for example, Young and Wilmott, 1962; Williamson, 1982; Bulmer, 1987; Etzioni, 1995). It has also been the subject of a range of policy initiatives, such as community care, community regeneration, and community safety, which have all made assumptions about the nature of the links between people who live in geographical proximity or who share characteristics or interests with each other. Often such policies have sought to encourage or enforce forms of behaviour based on normative assumptions about how people should relate to others. This is perhaps most evident in the policy of community care. This is based not only on a belief that older people, disabled people and those experiencing psychological distress should receive support 'in the community', rather than being segregated from the rest of society in long-stay institutions, but also on the assumption that care by family and friends is both the best and the preferred option in such circumstances (Barnes, 1997). There has not always been a close link between the analysis of community deriving from research, and the assumptions that have driven policy. In particular, the emphasis within official community care policy on family care not only conflated 'community' with 'family' as the source of support for individuals, but also largely failed to address the potential of communities to exclude those they regard as 'different'.

'Community' can be based on identity and interest as well as locality. Shared ethnicity, gender and sexuality can provide a basis for friendship, support and political action for people who may not primarily identify themselves in relation to the locality in which they live. Similarly, the 1980s and 1990s saw a substantial development of collective action among those who identify themselves as users of health and social care services, as disabled people, as survivors of psychological distress and/or of mental health services, or as carers. Disabled people, users ands survivors are working together to support each other and to achieve change within welfare services and in society more broadly. They draw on their collective experiences to propose action to overcome the barriers they face, and to provide support which enables community participation.

For those who have experienced stigma and exclusion, such 'communities of identity' can be more significant than a community defined by locality. Collective action of this type can also contribute to the diversity of identities which may be included within the population of any particular locality. Action which might be considered as 'community development' among people previously separated from 'ordinary life' in long-stay hospitals and residential units has been important not only in supporting disabled people and others to take part in community, but also in changing communities to enable that participation (Barnes, 1997).

USER MOVEMENTS

Collective action among disabled people and mental health service users has been theorized by reference to 'new social movements' (Barnes and Bowl, 2001; Campbell and Oliver, 1996; Shakespeare, 1993). Melucci (1985) has suggested that a shared identity 'constructed and negotiated through a repeated process of "activation" of social relationships connecting the actors' distinguishes 'new' from 'old' social movements. Identities are created and re-created not simply by 'being', but through action within such movements. New social movements are not solely or primarily concerned with redistribution, structural revolution or reform, as in the case of class-based movements, but with cultural and expressive objectives based on identity formation or consciousness raising (Cohen, 1985). Touraine (2000: 92) has described it in these terms: 'A social movement is never reducible to the defence of the interests of the dominated. Its ambition is always to abolish a relationship of domination, to bring about the triumph of a principle of equality, or to create a new society which breaks with the old forms of production, management and hierarchy.' The overarching objective can be expressed as one of transformation rather than restructuring and the means by which this is to be achieved is through a transformation of the values and meanings predominating in what has been variously termed the 'post-industrial' or 'post-modern' world.

We can see this in both the strategies and objectives of user groups. They seek change in the nature of health and social care services, and in the social policies which shape both the provision of welfare services and broader public policy. But their *underlying* objectives are concerned with transforming the way in which mental illness and disability are understood, and the way in which disabled people and people experiencing severe psychological distress are perceived. The methods they use to achieve this include user-led research and training, cultural expression and public awareness campaigns, as well as more direct involvement in policy-making.

There might be some reluctance among activists to define this as 'health promotion'. Within the disability movement there has been a powerful analysis of the inadequacy of the medical model and an assertion of the difference between illness and disability. Mental health service users and survivors have also challenged clinical perspectives on distress and madness. The motivation for action comes more from the experience of exclusion than of poor health. Where groups have organized around particular 'mental health problems', most notably in the case of the Hearing Voices movement (Romme and Escher, 1993), the aim has been to reclaim and redefine the meaning of such experiences, rather than to achieve a reduction in 'symptoms'.

Another dilemma in locating such action within the health promotion arena has been the response of some clinicians to user organization, particularly in the area of mental health. Constructions by clinicians of the purpose of 'user involvement' as *therapy* rather than *empowerment* have led to conflict (Barnes and Wistow, 1994), and expectations that users will conform to bureaucratic 'rules of the game' in the context of consultation or participation exercises have, in some cases, contributed to stress (Barnes and Bowl, 2001).

Nevertheless, both the process and outcome of such action can contribute to promoting health and well-being. They can achieve this directly as a result of the development of skills and the enhancement of self-esteem, and indirectly through producing more health-promoting services, and by contributing to the development of a more inclusive society. Models of health promotion which locate this within practices which have the aims of reducing inequalities and social exclusion, rather than of individual health improvement, are more consistent with the transformative objectives of user movements.

ACHIEVING CHANGE

Some examples will illustrate how user groups are pursuing their objectives and the issues they face in doing so. One of the longest established mental health user groups in the UK is the Nottingham Advocacy Group (NAG). NAG grew out of patients' meetings on hospital wards. It was strongly influenced by the Dutch user movement and has grown to become an umbrella organization for user groups within different service settings, advocacy projects and user representation within a wide range of decision-making fora in the city. Activists in NAG have played an important role in supporting the development of similar user-led initiatives elsewhere and in the formation of the UK Advocacy Network (UKAN) in 1991.

Interviews with NAG activists carried out for research in the early 1990s illustrated the importance of active involvement in such groups for the participants themselves, as well as the impact they achieved:

> In some ways it turned out to be a positive step for me. It changed my life around from something that was killing me, virtually, to something that I finally got some kind of reward in.
> ... it's given me a life and without it I wouldn't have dreamed of doing half the things I do now. It's given me confidence, assurance . . . I get up now and speak at a conference quite happily. A few years ago I would have no more done that than fly! So really we are here for ourselves as well as other people. (quoted in Barnes and Shardlow, 1996)

But the importance of this goes beyond individual personal development. Activists also spoke of the way in which their involvement in decision-making fora demonstrated that mental health service users, who are often regarded as incapable of decision-making on their own behalf, can play an important role in shaping policies and services. This impacts on wider perceptions of what it means to be someone with a mental health problem.

NAG has faced problems. While it is influential within the local mental health system, it has continually faced the problem of resourcing its work, and of persuading officials in all parts of the system that it has a role to play. There have also been differences of philosophy within the group: not all service users hold the same views about 'mental illness' nor about the priorities to be given to different strategies to support service users. One development initially under the NAG umbrella and later established as a separate initiative was 'Ecoworks'. Brian Davey, who played a key role in this, locates Ecoworks within the community development tradition (Davey, 1999). Its aim is to enable people who have used mental health services to become involved in small-scale work projects based on ecological principles. Rather than prioritizing changes in the mental health system, this initiative aims more directly to address social exclusion and the conditions which create this.

Elsewhere mental health service users, disabled people and others have become involved in user-led research which has the joint aims of exploring and disseminating users' views and of demonstrating the value of research in which users are fully represented in determining the subject matter and in carrying it out (e.g. Barnes and Mercer, 1997; Faulkner and Layzell, 2000). Others have become trainers and some are employed on postgraduate and professional training programmes, taking part in the education of professionals who will subsequently deliver services. Involvement in the process of knowledge production and dissemination is a potent demonstration of the challenge offered to traditional assumptions about professional knowledge and the power associated with it.

Older people constitute the largest group of people using community care and health services. Self-organization among older people is less developed than among other groups, but examples are emerging (for example, Barnes and Shaw, 2000; Cormie, 1999; Thornton and Tozer, 1995). Once again, studies of such experiences demonstrate the impact that collective action which values people's experiences can make on the individuals who take part: 'That's been one of the best things that's ever happened to me is getting to go there so that I could voice my opinion on things and say to them what I think. I feel, you feel you are getting somewhere by doing that and being able to do it, whereas before I couldn't' (Barnes and Bennet, 1998). But, as with the experience of mental health service users, the reluctance of some professionals to hear what users have to say, and the struggle to obtain the resources necessary to sustain and develop such initiatives, are never far away.

There is also a tendency among officials to construct the voices of service users as 'self-interested' and thus to question their legitimacy. Involvement in a user group *per se* is sometimes considered to mean that the users concerned are no longer 'representative' of the silent majority. The way in which people make their contributions can also be dismissed as 'over-emotional' or as expressing 'mere anecdotes' which do not have the same legitimacy as rational scientific argument. User organization has provided an important source of alternative knowledge and expertise and has produced real improvements for participants and the services they have sought to influence, but the balance of power is still firmly in favour of professionals.

NEW POLICY DIRECTIONS

The late 1990s saw important shifts in the construction of social problems and of policy responses to them. The identification of social exclusion as *the* problem for which social policy solutions were required marked official recognition that deprivation and inequality in material circumstances are associated with deprivation and inequality in terms of physical environments, educational and health status. There are three key aspects to this that are of central relevance to this discussion:

1   There is a changing focus from a service delivery to an issue or locality-based approach to policy-making.
2   There is an increasing focus on people as members of communities.
3   Communities are identified as deliverers of policy and creators of solutions as well as the context within which problems have to be understood. (For a longer discussion of this, see Barnes and Prior, 2000).

These changes should provide a more fertile environment within which user movements can play a role in challenging the social exclusion experienced by their members. In practical policy terms this will extend beyond the community care arena. It will take place within the context of Health Action Zones and Health Improvement Programmes as well as other locality-based initiatives to reduce social exclusion. For example, some HAZs have developed programmes focusing on mental health issues, on older people or on disabled people. The challenge will be to ensure that *locality*-based action to address the root causes of ill health can also include these groups, who have often found local communities to be unsupportive of the experiences of people regarded as 'different'.

3.3

COMMUNITY DEVELOPMENT AND HEALTH WORK IN NORTHERN IRELAND: CONTEXT, HISTORY AND DEVELOPMENT

Ruth Sutherland

How health is defined remains central to the business of health promotion. This is also true for 'community development', a dynamic concept meaning different things to different people according to time, place, culture and purpose. Community development, and community development and health work, in Northern Ireland (NI) have their own history, shaped by unique circumstances. In this contribution key issues in this history are highlighted and how they have shaped community development and health practice. In particular it is examined how, as a consequence of direct rule from London, the cleavage between state and citizen, the gap between policy and implementation, and poor infrastructure for health promotion, have constrained statutory health promotion from harnessing the energy of a vibrant voluntary and community sector. The contribution of the Community Development and Health Network is also described, and the current challenges for health and health promotion in NI are assessed. The aim is to show how difference can be an obstacle to collaboration, and how community development has potential in addressing health inequality and promoting health for all, despite these false divisions.

SOCIAL, ECONOMIC AND POLITICAL CONTEXT

The population of NI is small (about 1.6 million), geographically dispersed and disproportionately young, with a higher proportion of single parent households than mainland UK. In addition, NI is one of the poorest regions of the UK as measured by GDP per head, average incomes and the proportion of the population falling below the poverty thresholds (Wong and Morrissey, 1999), and has the highest unemployment rate of all UK regions. Long-term male unemployment (two years or more) is over twice that in the rest of the UK, so that NI has higher rates of reliance on state benefits than other UK regions, but also higher expenditure on food, fuel and clothing. Given this social and demographic context, the addition of what is euphemistically referred to as 'the Troubles' can only worsen an already poor health situation.

The three main causes of death in NI – heart disease, stroke and cancer –

hit the poorest in society first and worst (Gowdy, 1999). Comparisons between NI and western European countries show it to be below the European average life expectancy for men and considerably lower for women; for example, French women have an expectation of life more than five years longer than that of women in NI (Chief Medical Officer, 1999). As elsewhere, the most marginalized in NI endure the worst health: the average age at death for travelling people in Ireland is around the mid-forties – comparable with Third World statistics. Worse, there is evidence to show that 'people in disadvantaged groups not only suffer more ill health and die younger, but they are also less likely to receive or benefit from health and social care' (DHSS, 1996).

At the centre of 'the Troubles' lies the deep historical division created by religious, cultural and political differences, which has resulted in pervasive sectarianism. (For those unfamiliar with the term 'sectarianism', read racism: the process and the outcome are essentially the same.) Since 1969, the year which marked the height of the civil rights movement which sought universal suffrage and other moves toward equality, 3,601 people had been killed by 24 March 1998, and it is estimated that between 40,000 and 50,000 people had been injured (Smyth, 1998). In some years, this would have represented three Concorde tragedies each year in a population the size of a London borough, and scaled up to the UK population, it would represent 130,000 deaths (Bloomfield, 1998). The trauma has been protracted and some communities have suffered disproportionately. The dead have been predominately young men (91 per cent male, 37 per cent under 24 years and 53 per cent under 29 years) with the majority (53 per cent) being civilians, with no affiliation to the security forces or paramilitary organizations. The loss of life has been rather higher in the Catholic than in the Protestant population (Bloomfield, 1998). Civilian deaths are related to areas of deprivation, which tend to be disproportionately (though not exclusively) in Catholic communities.

Of course, mortality rates only reveal a fraction of the impact of conflict on health. Although deaths due to the conflict are predominately male, one might speculate that, like general health mortality and morbidity rates, while men die younger it is women – and, increasingly, children – who suffer in higher proportion (Smyth, 1998). This is important since women have dominated in peace building, and other community development and health activity. The strong women's movement, particularly in Belfast, has been a direct response by women to the conflict and has recently led to the formation of the Women's Coalition as a new political party. The growth of self-help and social support activity has become a vital community development and health action, in contrast to the common medical response of the 1970s – the liberal prescription of benzodiazepines (Valium and other tranquillizers).

There is a sense in which no one living in NI, even those who do not readily identify with either side of the sectarian divide, has escaped the impact of 'the Troubles'. The same is true at a policy level: debate and action on many health and social issues, such as poverty, unemployment, health inequalities or minority ethnic issues, have been overshadowed by this preoccupation. So, for example, NI has only been covered by race relations legislation since 1997, despite its diverse minority ethnic population which includes travelling people. Ironically, though, this impact has remained absent from the official and policy history of NI. In the past 30 years of regional health and social care strategy, the first mention of the impact of 'the Troubles' on health was in 1996 (DHSS, 1996). The first health and social services staff to work on post-traumatic stress disorder were sent to England in response to the British Midlands plane disaster in January 1989, while victims of trauma in NI were more or less left to support themselves (Bloomfield, 1998). This was a result of the 'business as usual' policy of the British government – not being seen to give into terrorism – and, together with the impact of direct rule, this confirmed the cleavage between state and citizen in NI which grew ever deeper as the conflict worsened.

These circumstances dictated that 'the Troubles' were not officially recognized: the official position permeated across statutory bodies and their workforce. The situation was compounded by the fact that many workers in the state sector did not come from the areas of greatest deprivation and worst violence. The collective collusion of these workers with the state's refusal to acknowledge the conflict might be seen as a way of coping with the chaos around them. The sectarian divisions within their own organizations also posed a problem, so that the only way to work together was to ignore the divisions and maintain a pretence of neutrality. Sectarian division in NI is often referred to as a 'glass curtain': you are never sure where it is, until you walk into it. It is certain that while the state workers of the time tried to present a position of neutrality – in the interests of staying alive – they were well aware of the sectarian divisions in the organizations and communities they worked in. It was commonplace for workers to use different names (either Catholic or Protestant) to fit in with different clients. In having to exclude themselves from the dominant political issue of conflict, state workers have also found themselves disengaged from other political health issues such as poverty and inequality.

Health promotion policy, like other social policy, was defined by Westminster. Civil service and statutory workers, with some exceptions, carried out central objectives and were supported and trained by British-based professional bodies and academic institutions. (A health promotion diploma and MSc, for example, were not available in NI for a long period, only being reinstated in 1992 at the University of Ulster.) On the whole, the link between community development and health promotion was not strong. Community development had been associated with social policy, particularly as a response to 'the Troubles', and traditionally health promotion was associated with the statutory sector and closely linked to medicine. Further, health promotion was constrained in developing a relationship with traditional allies such as local government and education, which might have brought it in closer contact with the experiences of local communities, particularly those most marginalized. Again, this was in part the result of direct rule, with local government responsibilities largely reduced to 'bins and burials' and education policy directed from Westminster. The well-known 'silo mentality' of government departments which do not communicate has been particularly marked in NI.

Yet as early as the late 1960s Maurice Hayes, the first director of the Community Relations Commission in NI, highlighted the value of community development and made the important point that religious tension was a symptom of an underlying social and economic disadvantage that needed to be tackled (Black, 1994). Much of the community development work in NI stemmed from the early community relations council, and it is clear that the community voluntary sector filled a social and economic vacuum. While political parties concentrated on constitutional matters, the voluntary and community sector focused on the impact of conflict on individuals, families and communities. Ironically, therefore, the long-term absence of democracy at local and regional level contributed to the development of a flourishing and increasingly sophisticated community and voluntary sector, although its activity has not always been recognized – even within the sector itself – as health-enhancing. Today, there are about 5,000 voluntary and community organizations in NI, 85 per cent of which have been founded since 1968. The sector is largely self-sustaining, with only a fifth of these organizations controlled from outside NI. Although many organizations are small (84 per cent have an annual turnover below £100,000), there are about 33,550 paid employees, accounting for 5 per cent of the NI workforce, alongside some 79,000 formal volunteers (NICVA, 1998). The role of the community/voluntary sector and community development was highlighted in the Good Friday Agreement, which saw their involvement as essential in supporting the emerging democratic and civil structures.

THE POLICY CONTEXT

Although much NI policy is dictated by Westminster, the need to work for equality and inclusion has required local innovation. Even during what have been referred to as 'the dark years', when community development activity in addressing health inequality was obliterated from government thinking, community development gained growing support in NI policy-making as a possible approach to addressing the social and health consequences of 'the Troubles'. In 1993, it gained a champion within the government office when the voluntary activity unit was established in the Department of Health and Social Services (more recently relocated to the new Department of Social Development). Despite the ebbs and flows, community development has been a more or less constant feature in NI since the 1930s (Logue, 1991). As elsewhere, health and social services face a crowded policy agenda, in which the theme of social justice has become important. Of course, this has a particular resonance in NI in the light of the established links between seeking peace and reconciliation, equity and inclusion through community development. Regional health strategy emphasizes the need for social justice as a central objective (DHSS, 1997a) and has defined community development at policy level:

> Community development is about strengthening and bringing about change in communities. It consists of a set of methods, which can broaden vision and capacity for social change and approaches, including consultation, advocacy and relationships with local groups. It is a way of working, informed by certain principles which seeks to encourage communities – people who live in the same areas or who have something in common – to tackle for themselves the problems which they face and identify to be important, and which empower them to change things by developing their own skills, knowledge and experience, and by working in partnerships with other groups and agencies. (DHSS, 1996)

This was regional health strategy before the election of a Labour government in 1997, which was later enhanced by the companion strategy *Well in 2000* (DHSS, 1997b) which set out new commitments. But although NI has an integrated health and social care structure, in practice the divisions are still rigid. Community development policy has become associated, in the DHSS, with social policy rather than health policy, and as a consequence, health promotion and social policy are separated. As an example, during the European Commission's third anti-poverty programme, of the 27 projects across Europe, only two or three developed a declared interest in health, and there was no link made at European level between the healthy cities movement and anti-poverty strategy. As a way of working, community development has become highly relevant to making health and social care more equitable and inclusive, but has had little impact on health promotion policy which continues to be narrowly defined.

Equality legislation, which is specific to NI and is a lynchpin of the Good Friday Agreement, provides a legislative framework for policy initiatives such as *Targeting Health and Social Need* and the need to promote good community relations. The legislation places a statutory duty on public authorities to have due regard to the need to promote equality of opportunity 'between persons of different religious belief, political opinion, racial group, gender, age, marital status, sexual orientation, ability' (Section 75 of the Northern Ireland Act 1998). In addition, authorities are required 'to have due regard to the desirability of promoting good relations between persons of different religious belief, political opinion or racial group'. There is also a statutory duty to consult: public bodies must set out strategies which specifically include those usually excluded in consultation. These new rights and responsibilities are designed to work for peace, and of course reconciliation and equality are key prerequisites for health. More recently there has also been a requirement that health and social services meet the needs of victims of 'the Troubles' (Bloomfield, 1998). This legislative context is very supportive to those involved in community development and health work.

COMMUNITY DEVELOPMENT AND HEALTH IN NI

The large and diverse community/voluntary sector in NI can trace its roots back to the 1930s, although an explicit link between community development and health was not made until the 1980s (Black, 1994). Two milestones in forging this link were the Moyard Health Profile (Ginnety et al., 1985) and the establishment of the Belfast healthy city project, both in 1985. Much more has followed, although there are few published accounts (DHSS, 1997a; DHSS Voluntary Activity Unit, 1999).

The Community Development and Health Network (CDHN) developed from informal contacts between people working on a range of community health projects across NI. These workers, from different sectors and perspectives, were motivated to come together for support and information exchange and, from early meetings in 1989, a number of common themes emerged. It was acknowledged that adopting a community development approach to health work presented a number of challenges, most importantly gaining credibility alongside 'mainstream' health promotion and health and social care; and how best to highlight specific health concerns such as inequalities in health, health rights and community health action, in the broader CD setting. At the macro level there were also concerns about the lack of an overall infrastructure for community health initiatives in NI, and the bias towards a medical model of health and health promotion which prioritized statutory body intervention and marginalized the inclusion of people and their communities in the identification, planning and delivery of actions to address health issues.

In order to begin to address these challenges – and as more and more people wanted to become involved in the network – funding was secured (in 1995) and a worker appointed (1996). In the five years since, organic growth has seen membership grow from about 35 to over 400, providing a firm foundation for the future (Kennedy, 1999). About three-quarters of members are from the voluntary/community sector, and one-quarter from the statutory sector. The network is a limited company and has established a charitable arm. Mindful of the need for independence, the network draws its funding from a wide range of sources.

The network defined a community development approach to health as: 'recognising the central importance of social support networks. It is a process by which a community defines its own health needs to bring about change. The emphasis is on collective action to redress inequalities in health and access to health care' (Black, 1994). The mission of the network is: 'to effect change at policy, organisational and practice level to promote and support community activity on health issues to promote action to redress poverty and inequalities in health.' One of the biggest challenges facing such a small organization continues to be how to develop such strategy and action at policy, organization and practice levels. Two examples of recent work show how CDHN has approached this challenge.

POLICY TO PRACTICE PILOT PROGRAMME

The 'Policy to Practice' initiative was a two-year action research project piloting a training, professional and organizational development programme to examine the enabling and constraining factors for statutory health and social services trusts in 'mainstreaming' CD approaches into their core business. It was developed in direct response to policy recommendations in the regional strategy and the mainstreaming document (DHSS Voluntary Activity Unit, 1999). Our motivation was to address the long-standing gap between policy and practice, and we set out with the intention of creating a dialogue with policy-makers to inform future development of community development policies. The project involved five community health and social services trusts, with staff at all levels being facilitated by a project manager from CDHN but managed within the trust. The programme was extensively evaluated using both internal self-evaluation and external objective assessment (reports of the process, evaluation and a training resource are available from CDHN).

The project generated valuable insights into the factors enabling and constraining the integration of community development approaches at policy, organizational and practice levels in the trusts. Many of the constraining factors related to structural issues or to 'custom and practice'. While the outcomes of 'policy to practice' are still unfolding, the project has created a role for the community/voluntary sector in policy development and training with statutory bodies, established CDHN as a credible project manager, and has led to a short secondment to a health and social services board to manage the development of their community development strategy (SHSSB, 2000).

TALES FROM THE FIELD

A second example is of research commissioned by CDHN which sought to set out what workers (paid or unpaid) in community development projects understand community development and health to be about. The report, 'Tales from the Field of Community Development and Health', highlights the strengths, opportunities, constraints and challenges of the work of 250 groups in NI (Ginnety, 2001). The work ranges from health information, health rights, self-help and social support, community education and community action on health issues to campaigning and partnership working, and would otherwise be unrecognized. CDHN is now working to respond to the needs expressed in the report with a resource manual to support those working in the field.

CONCLUSION

I have presented a brief overview of the complex history of community development and health work in NI. The widespread community development activity in NI demonstrates enormous potential for health promotion if the division between statutory health promotion and community/voluntary sector activity can be bridged, and shows the important contribution that can be made by people and their communities to their own health.

Finally, what are the key challenges which face future health promoters in NI? First, peace and political stability: we have an imperfect peace and precarious fledgling political institutions. The business of making democracy work is not easy, yet vital to the health of our population. Second, devolution: the impact that devolution might have on the current policy framework has to be accepted as the price of working for democracy. It has taken a long time to get issues relating to poverty and ill-health on the government agenda, and it is frustrating that policies made at a local level may well prove less radical, due to the generally conservative values of our political parties and to some extent our society. We can hope that with peace will come renewed, open and informed public debates on social policy. Devolution will also challenge the community/voluntary sector to adapt to new roles and new institutions. Can participatory democracy thrive and develop alongside representative democracy? If the policy vacuum disappears, can the sector adjust? And will the Northern Ireland Assembly accommodate?

Third, progress also depends on whether the equality agenda is successfully implemented, since huge expectations now surround the equality legislation. Fourth, the ability and motivation of statutory organizations to change: new resources are expected to be consumed by the acute sector, and although our work has influenced statutory health promotion strategy in a limited way, it remains dominated by individual and lifestyle approaches to health promotion. Finally, there is the question of whether the community/voluntary sector can act strategically and collaboratively, given the inevitable shrinkage of the sector as EU funding linked to our previous 'objective one status' now begins to fall.

4

SOCIAL EXCLUSION, DISCRIMINATION AND THE PROMOTION OF HEALTH

Maria Duggan

Tackling health inequality and combating social exclusion are central themes in New Labour's public health policy. This chapter reviews some of the evidence and theories of how poverty, disadvantage and discrimination affect health and considers the implications for health promotion. It argues that certain groups of people are politically excluded from the conditions required to create and sustain health. This suggests that there are two key challenges for health promotion. The first is to define a model of health which demonstrates the relevance of, and linkages between biological, behavioural, psychosocial, economic and environmental determinants of health. The second is to put this model into practice by developing strategies that can assist individuals, groups and communities in challenging the complex personal and social factors that exclude them from good health.

SOCIAL EXCLUSION

Social exclusion is a shorthand term for what can happen when people or areas suffer from a combination of problems such as unemployment, poor skills, low incomes, poor housing or homelessness, high crime environments, bad health and family breakdown. In the past, governments have tried to deal with each of these problems individually, but there has been little progress in tackling the complicated links between them, or preventing them from arising in the first place. People who are socially excluded suffer multiple disadvantages which impact on health. The evidence set out below suggests that the social exclusion of individuals and groups is as much a cause as a consequence of poor health. If so, it follows that strategies for removing barriers to social participation, and addressing the multiple disadvantages of social exclusion, must be among the goals of health promoting activity.

CONTEXT

Many developed countries saw changes in income-related policies during the period from the 1970s to the late 1990s, with a range of attempts to constrain the social welfare system. During the same period, a number of countries saw a growth in adverse health effects, with those in the UK being particularly severe. There is evidence suggesting that a robust social welfare system protects against worsening public health, even in times of deep economic recession (Mackenbach and Droomers, 1999). The growth in poverty and the erosion of the welfare state in the UK during this period are directly implicated in the widening health gap and the social exclusion of large numbers of individuals and communities.

The 1979–97 period of Conservative government in the UK was one of rapidly widening inequality. Average real incomes grew between 1979 and 1996, but this increasing national prosperity was achieved at the cost of widening income inequality and a sharp rise in the proportion of households below the EC decency threshold (less than 50 per cent of average income). The number of people living below this threshold more than doubled from the beginning of the 1980s to the mid-1990s. At a time when overall average income grew by 40 per cent, the incomes of the poorest 20 per cent of the population were little or no higher in real terms (Hills, 1998).

Underlying this increasing inequality in income and living standards has been a deeper process of socio-economic polarization. As in other EC countries, the rate of unemployment in the UK increased in this period, which was associated with rapid changes in the pattern of employment. There was an increase in two-earner households and no earner households, polarizing both employment and housing tenure, with no-earner households living in social housing (in state-provided or state-subsidized housing) and a growth in homelessness.

During the same period there was a significant change in population health, with a marked growth in health inequality. The health of Britain today is probably better than ever before: death rates have been falling steadily since the start of the twentieth century and life expectancy at birth has risen from 44 years for men and 48 years for women in the 1890s, to almost 75 for men and 80 for women in the 1990s. Infant death, commonly used as an indicator of a nation's health, has fallen from around 150 deaths for every 1000 births per year to approximately 8 per 1000 today. But while the overall picture is one of relative health and affluence, there are stark and increasing differences in health between different groups of people and different parts of the country. Why does such health inequality occur, and why is it so pronounced in the UK compared with other developed countries?

NATIONAL TRENDS IN HEALTH INEQUALITIES

Trends in health inequalities have been well documented in recent years. Current concerns can be traced back to Tudor Hart's 'inverse care law' in 1971, which drew attention to the fact that the provision of high quality health care tended to be lowest in areas where the need for it was the greatest (Hart, 1971). Increasing concern led to a series of investigations, most notably the Black Report, commissioned in 1977 by a Labour government but ignored by the Conservative government when it was published in 1980. It took almost another 20 years before the government acknowledged the need to address health inequalities, even though the term itself was not used and could only be spoken about as the euphemism 'health variations'. In the 20 years since the publication of the Black Report a wide range of research has confirmed that health inequalities in the UK are not only persistent but increasing. The most recent publication, the Acheson inquiry, provides clear evidence of the persistence of inequalities in health (Acheson, 1998). Despite recent changes to the tax and benefits system, the difference in life expectancy between male unskilled and professional workers increased from 5.5 years in 1972 to 9.5 years in 1996 (ONS, 1999).

WHAT IS HEALTH?

There is a long and rich history of attempts to define health, and although there has long been an acceptance of the social nature of health, there has been little effort to respond with policies which accept the interconnectedness of a range of social, economic, environmental, biological and behavioural factors. Two well-known models of health are those of Whitehead (1995) and Labonte (1998).

Layers of influence

Dahlgren and Whitehead propose a model built on 'layers of influence, one on top of the other' (see Figure 4.1). In this model, the inner core consists of factors that are 'fixed' and not modifiable (age, sex and hereditary factors) with surrounding layers which can, in principle, be modified. Individual 'lifestyle' factors are those that govern health-related behaviour and choices, but since individuals interact with a wider group of family, friends and communities their choices and behaviours are influenced by these. More pervasive influences on health are located in the layer of living and working conditions, which govern access to essential commodities, resources and services. Overarching all of these layers are socio-economic, cultural and environmental conditions, which bear down on every other layer. Whitehead notes:

> It is the range and inter-relationship of all the different determinants of health that [the] figure ... seeks to address. If one health hazard or risk factor is focused upon, it is important to examine how it fits with the other layers of influence, and whether it could be considered a primary cause or merely a symptom of a larger problem represented in the other layer ... In thinking about a policy response, questions need to be asked about the size of the contribution each of the four layers and their constituent factors make to the health divide (between different socio-economic groups); the feasibility of changing specific factors; and the complementary action that would be required to influence linked factors in other layers. (Whitehead, 1995: 24)

Figure 4.2 below describes a socio-ecological model of health developed by the Federal Canadian Heart Health Initiative and the Toronto Health Department. The World Health Organisation has subsequently adopted the model. In this model, the key determinants are identified as 'risk conditions', defined as those living and working conditions that are affected by political and economic decisions and forces. Labonte points out: 'These conditions are

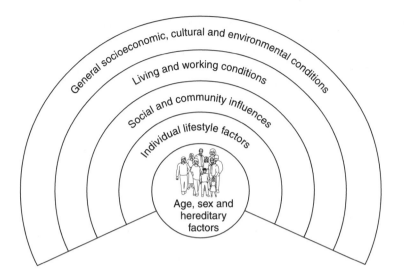

Figure 4.1 The main determinants of health
Source: Dahlgren and Whitehead (1991), Figure 1

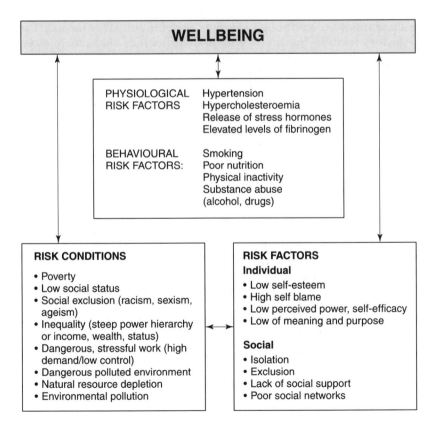

Figure 4.2 Socio-ecological model of health
Source: Labonte (1998)

unequally distributed by virtue of being conditions of comparative inequality' (1998: 7). Risk conditions increase the relative risk of ill health and early death directly, and also through the psychosocial risk factors experienced by individuals. In this model, perceptions of low social status and lack of power increase both the likelihood of sickness (the physiological risk factors) and of unhealthy lifestyle (the behavioural risk factors), particularly smoking, poor nutrition, physical inactivity and substance abuse. All of these factors are likely to be intensified in those who are socially excluded.

WHY DOES INEQUALITY AFFECT HEALTH?

Although the available research illuminates theoretically how health inequalities are the outcome of interlocking layers of influence which are influenced by the socio-economic structure, it almost invariably demonstrates how the underlying influences manifest themselves in home and work environments and in the daily habits and routines of life. As a result, we know much more about the effects of factors close to the individual than we do about factors which are close to the social structure. Among the individual influences, attention has focused on material, psychosocial and behavioural factors. Material factors include the physical environment of the home and workplace, together with living standards secured through earnings, benefits and other income. Psychosocial factors include the life events and difficulties that create stress for individuals and families, and the social networks and supportive relationships that enable people to meet these difficulties. Among behavioural factors, diet, exercise and smoking have all been singled out. These proximate influences cluster together: for example, an individual in poverty and poor housing is likely also to be disadvantaged in access to social support and is more likely to have health-damaging habits like cigarette smoking.

Psychosocial factors affecting health

Recently, increasing attention has focused on the strength of psychosocial influences on health. It has long been understood that the impact of stressful life events, such as bereavement, increased the risk of ill health or even premature death (Rees and Lutkins, 1967), but it took a series of factory closures in the 1960s and 1970s to demonstrate that psychosocial factors might be important contributors to health inequalities. Studies at that time showed that health deteriorated when people became insecure and not only when they knew that there were going to be redundancies (Cobb and Kasl, 1977). These findings are reinforced by others which indicate that social support and sense of control are also closely associated with health (Brunner and Marmot, 1999). Increasing evidence suggests that anything contributing to chronic anxiety is likely to worsen health in a grossly unequal society like our own. This evidence may have particular relevance for our understanding of the health consequences of social exclusion. This research underpins and reinforces the models of health discussed above. Labonte argues:

Because people caught in this 'web' of risk conditions and risk factors experience less social support and greater isolation, they are often less likely to be
active in community groups or processes concerned with improving risk
conditions in the first place. This 'feedback loop' reinforces isolation and self
blame reinforcing the experience of disease/dis-ease. (Labonte, 1998)

Social cohesion and health

More equal societies appear to be more socially cohesive and healthier. Richard
Wilkinson suggests that:

The combination of increasing social status differentials and deteriorating
social relations could hardly be a more potent mix for population health.
Social status and social support or social affiliation are – at least in the developed world – perhaps the two most important risk factors for health. Both
have been associated with two, three or even fourfold differences in mortality. (Wilkinson, 1996)

Wilkinson attributes the better health of people living in more egalitarian societies to the greater cohesiveness of such societies. Research from several sources
lends support to this idea. Putnam notes that his 'index of civic community' (a
way of measuring the strength of people's involvement in the community) was
closely correlated with income inequality (Putnam et al., 1993). Putnam notes
that 'civic' communities and regions are characterized by 'distaste for hierarchi-
cal authority patterns' and suggests that 'political leaders in the civic regions are
far more enthusiastic supporters of political equality than their counterparts in
less civic regions'. Similarly, Kawachi and others found that people were likely
to feel more trustful towards others in those US states in which income differentials were smaller (Kawachi et al., 1997). Other studies suggest that violent
crime and homicide are highest where income differentials are greatest (Hsieh
and Pugh, 1993).

This accumulated research indicates that inequality has an adverse
impact on everyone's health and that those at the bottom suffer most, through
the interaction of a range of material factors with psychosocial factors. In particular, they endure low levels of self-esteem and high levels of 'social anxiety',
which is bad for health (Davey Smith, 1996; Macleod et al., 1999). If this is
accepted, it follows that the rapid growth in income inequality in the UK from
the 1970s to the late 1990s, and the growth of other forms of disadvantage and
social exclusion, are directly implicated in causing and sustaining the growth
of health inequalities during the same period. Narrowing the health gap therefore requires action to tackle social exclusion. This may well mean the
development of strategies that utilize a range of social and environmental
interventions such as regeneration and employment schemes, benefits campaigns and community development. It will also mean the involvement of a
wide range of statutory and voluntary agencies and of people who may be
socially excluded.

SOCIAL CAPITAL

The concept of 'social capital' is relevant to the task facing health promotion specialists and others tackling health inequalities and social exclusion. The concept currently occupies a prominent place in the debate over the government's social policy programme – even though, like the 'third way', its exact nature remains unclear. In particular, the difference between social capital and social cohesion – a broad umbrella term lacking clear theoretical meaning – remains to be clarified. Higher social capital, it is suggested, is implicated in a range of positive policy outcomes, including higher rates of economic growth, lower crime rates, better local and national government and better public health. It is suggested that it is a valuable way of understanding the causes of the growing gap in health status between rich and poor, and for the development of public health interventions aimed at improving the health of the poorest.

Defining social capital

There are many different definitions of social capital in use. The concept involves social relationships, social support, formal and informal social networks, group membership, shared norms, trust, reciprocity and community and civic engagement (Coleman, 1988; Etzioni, 1995; Fukuyama, 1995; Putnam et al., 1993). Putnam has written most widely on social capital and defines it as the 'features of social organization such as networks, norms and social trust that facilitate co-ordination and collaboration for mutual benefit' (Putnam, 1995). Social capital links the individual with institutions and organizations through social and civic networks. Active participation in such networks builds the social trust that underpins cohesiveness and collaboration, the important resources for health and health creation (Brehm and Rahn, 1997). The idea of social capital therefore places a high value on co-operation, participation and social inclusion.

The value of social capital to health improvement strategies

It has been argued that the idea of social capital has a role to play in improving and sustaining the health of the public, in three ways. First, it emphasizes the importance of social approaches to public health and health promotion. Second, it suggests that social capital can act as a buffer against the worst effects of deprivation. And third, it focuses attention on the important contribution that formal and informal social and civic networks and skills can make to the health of populations, and thus provides renewed impetus to collective, collaborative community-based public health efforts to reduce inequalities and reinforces partnership and participatory approaches to promote health.

Although studies designed to specifically measure the relationship between social capital and health are sparse, such evidence as we have appears to point to the existence of an association. For example:

- A 20-year study of governance and wealth production in Italy found that levels of social capital were related to life expectancy and infant mortality (Putnam et al., 1993).

- A study of professional men found that those with the lowest level of social networks and group membership were more likely to die from cardiovascular disease, accidents and suicide (Kawachi et al., 1996).
- A study of deprived children compared those who were 'doing well' or thriving developmentally with those who were not. The presence of any single social capital indicator increased the likelihood of a child doing well by 27 per cent; any two increased it by 66 per cent. The important indicators were perception of personal social support, actual support within neighbourhoods and church membership (Runyan et al., 1998).
- Certain preventive activities, such as seeking screening, are significantly related to levels of social capital in women engaged in peer networking activities and outreach education. Local advocacy activities, campaigning for rights, encouraging people to vote in local elections and the development of new social networks, are also related to high levels of social capital (Higgins et al., 1996).
- A study of 480 householders in Luton demonstrated a significant relationship between levels of health and aspects of social capital. It compared a disadvantaged area with good health to one with poor health, allowing an assessment of whether or not social capital and its indicators might be different in different contexts, and began to explore how social capital, if it existed as a coherent set of processes, might affect health (Campbell et al., 1998).

This last study suggests that it is not simply the *existence* of social networks but their *nature* that is important in health terms. They need to be outward-looking and engaged with the wider community, and in their absence it seems unlikely that local services will be used. This may be of particular significance in the understanding of the ways in which social exclusion affects health. Other studies shed further light on this issue. In families in particular hardship, the capacity to engage in wider social and civic life is greatly reduced (Moser, 1996), and the inevitable preoccupation with family survival focuses activities within the family but, paradoxically, this may lead to further disadvantage. Forming relationships with the outside world builds confidence, access to services and support, a sense of greater control, and promotes social inclusion. Even strong inward-looking networks do not necessarily do so. On the basis of this evidence, the idea of social capital provides us with a new set of indicators for measuring community-based interventions for health. Just as important, it legitimizes a range of interventions aimed at improving health by bolstering local networks and encouraging participation in local life and using local services and facilities.

The limitations of social capital

Some argue that the link between social support, social networks, self-efficacy and good health has been known for some time (Wadsworth, 1996), so how does the notion of social capital develop our current understanding or offer a fresh perspective to health promoters? One answer is to suggest that if inequalities in health are indeed driven by relative power imbalances in societies, then the concept of social capital provides one way of understanding the problem and paves the way for an approach to improving health that incorporates community empowerment goals. Effectively involving local people in shaping and influencing decision-making about health, and enabling sustained involvement, increases social capital at local level. This kind of participation in the civic structures of local life is precisely the kind of outward-looking networking which the available research suggests will have positive health outcomes.

Set against this, some commentators have suggested that, whatever the value of legitimizing a community empowerment approach to improving health, the paucity of current evidence and the imprecision of the idea of social capital demand a critical perspective (Hunter, 1998). Hunter suggests that social capital can mean many things to many people, appealing both to social democrats and neo-liberals. For the former, the concept supports the case for renewed efforts at 'social engineering', using the state to nurture and sustain social capital at a local level; while for the latter, it encourages 'rolling back the state', asserting that big government is bad, and arguing that individuals are disempowered. So, in a neo-liberal political context, social capital may divert attention from the causes of inequality onto its effects. As one commentator argues: 'Income inequalities are neither necessary nor inevitable. Moreover, understanding the contextual causes of income inequality may also influence our notion of the causal pathways involved in inequality-health status relationships (and vice versa)' (Coburn, 2000).

Labonte is similarly critical, arguing that 'social capital . . . allows elites who benefit from economic practices that undermine social cohesion to voice that loss without necessarily linking it back to those practices that privilege them' (1999). Whether or not the concept is a smokescreen which obscures our analysis of the root causes of inequality, it is worth noting that even early proponents of social capital (particularly Robert Putnam) are now not so sure about the sustainability of social capital in communities where it has previously been shown to be strong. For instance, in his recent discourse on the disappearance of civic America, Putnam pins the blame firmly on television (Putnam, 1995) which, in his view, is the destroyer of strong social capital and has done more than any other development over the past 40 years to loosen the ties of strong civic association.

At present, therefore, our expectations of social capital both as an explanatory construct and as a goal of health promoting activity should be modest. It is not possible, given the current state of the evidence, to make an unequivocal connection between social capital and public health. It is also true that many of the assumptions underpinning social capital need to be examined more rigorously than they have been previously. But, of course, none of this means that a community empowerment approach to health improvement is invalid.

POLICY IMPLICATIONS

Ultimately, the key to tackling health inequalities and promoting social inclusion lies in narrowing the income gap between rich and poor and in transforming the unequal power relations which characterize our society. This requires an effective assault on the long-term causes of poverty such as unemployment and low pay, as well as building the skills and capacity of individuals to engage in fulfilling work and to participate in society. The evidence suggests, in particular, that polices must address child poverty and improving welfare services such as social housing, social services, public transport and community health services, all of which are used disproportionately by poor households and enhance the capacity for social inclusion.

Further, much more redistribution of income is needed. As the Acheson Report and others have demonstrated, many of those in poverty cannot work. If they are to keep up with the rest of society then redistribution, whether through benefits or tax credits, will have to increase. And, finally, we must broaden the attention of policy from poverty, deprivation and social exclusion to society as a whole. We need to face up to the central message of the research, which is that we cannot hope to 'cure' inequalities in health in isolation, as if they were independent of the wider social structure that generates them. This will, inevitably, involve policies that challenge the dominant values of our current social and political system by enabling and supporting greater participation in the political process by those who are currently excluded from it.

4.1

ANTI-POVERTY STRATEGIES

Pete Alcock

RESPONDING TO POVERTY

Poverty is a complex social problem, as we saw in Chapter 4 (see also Alcock, 1997). It overlaps with social exclusion, is defined in both absolute and relative terms, and is measured in both quantitative and qualitative ways. Inevitably, then, not all commentators agree on what poverty is, or on how much poverty there is in the UK today. However, they do all agree on one thing: whatever poverty is, it is a *problem* – and it is a problem which requires a social policy response. We should be seeking to remove, or reduce, the problem of poverty through policy development and policy intervention; hence the importance for social policy of anti-poverty policies, or strategies.

The problem of poverty contains two important, and different, dimensions however. First, poverty is a social – or structural – phenomenon. The existence of poverty in a wealthy country such as the UK means that some people are struggling to survive and to participate in modern life. This should be a matter of moral concern to us all but it is also a matter of social concern. The existence of poverty undermines social cohesion and social order and, in extreme circumstances, may be a contributory cause of crime, disorder and unrest. It is therefore in our collective interest to reduce or remove poverty.

Second, poverty is an individual – or experiential – phenomenon. People who are poor experience real hardship and deprivation and they need support and assistance to cope with these pressures. Even where poor people may not demand assistance – and there is growing understanding of why poor people do not always promote their own cause vigorously (see Beresford et al., 1999) – it is widely recognized that policy intervention should seek to provide help. So anti-poverty policy also aims to provide particular support to poor people.

Clearly, anti-poverty policies must seek to address both the individual and the collective dimensions of the problem of poverty. There have been traditionally disputes over the importance to be accorded to these two dimensions of the problem of poverty, as well as over the kinds of policy interventions which are appropriate responses to each of them. Some anti-poverty policies have emphasized collective, and others individual, approaches and there have occasionally been conflicts, or contradictions, between the different types of policy which have followed from each.

In terms of overall expenditure, and the number of people affected, the social security system is by far the most significant anti-poverty policy in the UK today. Over £100bn a year in social security benefits is distributed to over half of the population. Although many benefit recipients are not poor – for instance, child benefit and pensions are paid on the basis of age, not need – a significant part of the social security system does aim directly at the relief of poverty. This is particularly true of means tested benefits. These draw on the Poor Law legacy of the nineteenth century to target a basic minimum income to those who can show, through a means-test, that they are unable to provide for themselves. The aim of these benefits, in particular, is to redistribute resources from the 'rich' to the poor in order to reduce individual hardship, and to promote social cohesion by ensuring that society guarantees a minimum standard of living for all.

There is much debate about the extent to which means-tested and other social security benefits are appropriate vehicles for redistributing resources and relieving poverty, and there is considerable evidence that in practical terms they do not always succeed in reaching all of those who might need, or be entitled to, them (see McKay and Rowlingson, 1999). Nevertheless, social security remains the main instrument of anti-poverty action in the UK and in most other developed nations.

However, it is not the only instrument. Because social security does not always reach all those for whom it is intended, and because it does not always provide sufficient support for those experiencing particular hardships, there has been much criticism by academic researchers of its efficacy as an anti-poverty strategy, beginning with the seminal work by Abel Smith and Townsend in 1965. In particular, there is a growing body of research evidence which suggests that social security policies have not been able to address the income inequalities that are associated with poor health. From the Black Report (Townsend and Davidson, 1982) of the 1980s to the Acheson Inquiry (1998) of the 1990s, official reports have confirmed growing inequalities in health in the UK. Research by Wilkinson (1996) has suggested that greater inequality in a society is associated with higher levels of illness and early death. Continuing poverty is therefore a problem of poor health too – although this is generally overlooked, or ignored, in medical models of health promotion, which emphasize lifestyle choices rather than structural inequalities.

The limitations of social security policies led in the last quarter of the twentieth century to the development of alternative policies to combat poverty based not upon broad strategies for the redistribution of resources, but rather upon focused, or targeted, activities to help individual poor people or the communities in which they lived. It is these alternative policies which are usually referred to as 'anti-poverty strategies', and they have become much more widespread within policy planning at the beginning of the twenty-first century. They have also, to a limited extent, taken on the specific aim of weakening the link between poverty and poor health.

LOCAL ANTI-POVERTY ACTION

Anti-poverty strategies generally target their assistance through a geographical focus on areas where research evidence suggests that poverty is particularly concentrated. This is, in part, a result of the (inevitably) limited resources available for anti-poverty work but it is also the product of a belief that 'local' action can work with poor people within their communities to challenge the factors that contribute to poverty and exclusion. Such focused activity has obvious attractions, but it also brings some important problems. These can be summarized as:

- *Boundary disputes* – a local focus inevitably involves drawing boundaries around the areas to be helped, and these will result in arbitrary cut-off points. A boundary will exclude many poor people who live outside the area, yet include many non-poor people within it. This is also likely to bias activity towards urban areas, where poverty is concentrated, rather than rural areas, where it is dispersed yet may be more severe.
- *Negative labelling* – focusing activity on particular areas involves identifying them as highly deprived. This may not be welcomed by local policy-makers – or local people.
- *Picking winners* – most local policy initiatives are expected to result in observable improvements in local circumstances, since policy intervention should make a difference. This means that areas, and projects, are more likely to be selected where change can be more easily achieved. This may not benefit those in most need, for whom real improvements will take time and may require other social and economic changes.
- *Blaming the victim* – local anti-poverty strategies focus upon 'helping poor people to help themselves', which carries an implication that it is only what local people are doing, or not doing, which leads to their poverty; and ignores the broader social and economic forces which may have caused local deprivation (for instance, factory closure). This can lead to the assumption that the poor are to blame for their poverty and need to change their ways to escape from it. Many local anti-poverty projects have recognized that this is not the case (see Community Development Project, 1977), yet local anti-poverty activity cannot change wider social circumstances.

Current policy initiatives to combat poverty at a local level can largely be traced back to the central government programmes promoted in the late 1960s and early 1970s, in part as a response to the criticisms of social security policy made by commentators such as Abel Smith and Townsend. These activities were modelled on similar programmes developed in the United States as part of its so-called 'War on Poverty' (Higgins, 1978; James, 1970), and included the Education Priority Areas (EPA) and the Community Development Projects (CDP), mentioned above.

Despite the many innovative and adventurous activities sponsored by these programmes, however, government support for them was short-lived, with EPAs and CDPs lasting less than ten years. The most significant was the Urban Programme, which provided support for a range of neighbourhood projects, if additional funding was also provided by the relevant local authority. This encouraged local authorities to become involved in community projects and continued until this partnership funding was replaced by the Single Regeneration Budget (SRB) in the early 1990s. In the 1970s and 1980s local authorities also began to take on responsibility for some of the innovative local projects begun in the national programmes, in particular the welfare rights and advocacy work pioneered in the CDPs (Bradshaw, 1975).

Welfare rights work had emerged in the 1970s as a key feature of local anti-poverty action. Rights and advocacy work with local claimants revealed that many of them were not getting the social security and other welfare benefits to which they might be entitled and that, by helping them to secure these rights, the incomes and living standards of claimants could be enhanced. Many local authorities began to employ welfare rights workers and support local voluntary agencies providing advice and assistance to local citizens (Berthoud et al., 1986). Although this work was in part driven by a desire to improve local social services (many welfare rights workers were employed in social work departments), it was clear that it had a significant anti-poverty dimension.

In the 1980s, in particular, this anti-poverty profile became of greater concern to a number of councils, notably the large, Labour-controlled, metropolitan authorities who were voicing strong opposition to the public service cuts being imposed by the then Conservative government under Margaret Thatcher. Authorities such as Sheffield, Newcastle and the Greater London Council (GLC) soon expanded their support for welfare rights into a broader range of actions to combat local poverty and challenge central government. These included employment protection and creation, and subsidized local transport (notably the GLC's 'Fares Fair' campaign), and they were increasingly presented as part of a local *strategy* to combat poverty.

Local strategies to combat poverty were all the more significant in the 1980s because, during this period, central government dismissed claims that poverty continued to be a problem in late twentieth-century Britain and argued instead that government activity should focus upon the promotion of wealth (see especially the speech by Moore, 1989). This inevitably brought central and local government into conflict, and resulted in tighter restrictions on local authority activity and, in the case of the GLC, outright abolition. Nevertheless the scale of local anti-poverty activity continued to grow and in the 1990s it extended beyond the bigger metropolitan boroughs to include large numbers of councils of all kinds throughout the UK (see Alcock et al., 1995).

Despite the lack of central government support for local anti-poverty action, support did develop in the 1980s from the supra-national agencies of the European Union. EU programmes for regional development (ERDF) and social regeneration (ESF) provided resources for local projects to renew infrastructure and promote education and training in deprived areas, including many areas in Britain. The EU also supported three programmes to combat poverty and social exclusion, which provided temporary funding for pilot projects on local anti-poverty action, including a small number of projects in the UK. These 'poverty programmes' were discontinued in 1994, in part at the request of the UK government, but the development and training programmes have continued.

Of course, despite the evident commitment and innovation of many of these new anti-poverty initiatives, the structural limitations of local action remained. Local anti-poverty action did not lead to any significant redistribution of resources towards poor people, and indeed broader inequalities grew dramatically worse during the 1980s and early 1990s (Hills, 1995). In part, this was a product of national and international economic forces and in part a result of the economic priorities of national policy; but whatever the cause, it significantly undermined the efforts and achievements of local anti-poverty action.

What is more, although local authority anti-poverty action included a wide range of initiatives across areas such as social security, housing, employment and transport, health improvement and health promotion did not feature widely in these activities – despite the continuing growth of inequalities in health, discussed above and explored recently by Shaw et al. (1999). This neglect of an explicit health focus may have been the result of relatively poor relations between local authorities and a National Health Service which was driven by different priorities, but it was also a product of the lack of knowledge of health issues among some anti-poverty activists. Nevertheless a wide range of anti-poverty projects focusing directly upon poor health and health inequalities did develop in the 1980s and early 1990s, and these were catalogued in some detail by Laughlin and Black in 1995. More recently, initiatives promoted by the Labour government since 1997 have been able to draw on the experiences and innovations of these projects.

ANTI-POVERTY STRATEGIES IN THE TWENTY-FIRST CENTURY

Central government policies towards local anti-poverty action had, in fact, begun to change in the early 1990s under the Major government. Although not presented as anti-poverty initiatives, the new programmes for City Challenge and SRB did encourage a new partnership between central and local government in the identification and implementation of local action to promote economic and social regeneration. SRB in particular provided support for a new range of local projects targeted directly towards areas of high social deprivation and aiming to achieve change across a range of social and economic dimensions.

The election of the new Labour government in 1997 saw the major acceleration of such partnership activity, together with the rapid promotion of a wide range of new programmes to combat poverty and social exclusion through local action. Perhaps the most significant change here, however, was the recognition by the Labour government of the continuing, and escalating, problem of poverty. Labour was keen to resurrect the 'p-word', and to add to it a commitment to address the broader problem of social exclusion – revealed most clearly in the 1999 report *Opportunity for All* (Department of Social Security, 1999) which included a list of 32 indicators of poverty and social exclusion against which the achievement of new government policies would be measured annually.

Much of Labour's strategy for combating poverty and exclusion focused on the promotion of employment opportunities through the 'Welfare to Work' programme. This included changes to social security benefits for those on low wages, a national minimum wage, and the 'New Deal' to provide training and work experience for the young unemployed (and later, other groups too). However, the government also continued and expanded the SRB programme, and established a range of other central government initiatives to promote local action, including employment, education and health action zones. Health Action

Zones (HAZs) signified a new departure in the promotion of local heath gain through partnership action between local authorities, health authorities and other key local agencies. HAZs provided a focus, and a legitimacy, for the local project action described earlier by Laughlin and Black (1995) – in particular, the development by health workers of initiatives to combat the broader structural causes of poor health and the promotion of partnership working with other statutory and voluntary agencies.

Within the first year of office Tony Blair also established a high profile Social Exclusion Unit (SEU), responsible directly to the Cabinet Office. The SEU did not have a significant budget for anti-poverty action but it did include officers from a wide range of government departments and external agencies, and it was charged with the pursuit of 'joined-up' solutions to designated problems of social exclusion. The most important was the concentration of local poverty revealed in the SEU's major report on neighbourhood renewal in 1998. This resulted in a further new policy initiative, the 'New Deal for Communities', which established additional anti-poverty projects in 17 'pathfinder' local areas, since followed by more.

At the beginning of the twenty-first century, therefore, local anti-poverty action in the UK is at its most vibrant and widespread. For the first time, central and local government are working together to promote local anti-poverty strategies (with continuing EU support), and the range of programmes and policies now in operation is greater than at any time in the past. Local anti-poverty action is now promoted in many other advanced industrial nations, most notably in many other EU member states where similar programmes to those in the UK are underway. Health improvement is obviously a key element of the work of the Health Action Zones; but it is also increasingly a part of the broader activities included in local authority anti-poverty strategies or the projects supported by programmes such as the New Deal for Communities.

Of course, local anti-poverty strategies are exactly that, and continue to carry with them all the conflicts and contradictions of local action, as outlined above. Much has already been achieved by local projects and local initiatives to combat poverty, but there are inevitable limitations within the local approach. Unless local action is located within a broader national, and international, strategy for tackling poverty and promoting economic and social regeneration, much of the depth and breadth of local poverty will remain unchanged, and perhaps unchallenged. So although local anti-poverty strategies are now an important part of social policy planning, they are only a part.

4.2

DISABILITY AND PUBLIC HEALTH

Lorraine Gradwell

Can disabled people enjoy good health, or are we necessarily and inherently unhealthy? Can public health professionals support the attainment of health, or does the presence of impairment, disease or debilitating conditions preclude a healthy lifestyle and a sense of well-being? What *is* health, in relation to disabled people?

It is accepted that not only is good health about an optimum level of physical and mental well-being, but also about enjoying an appropriate lifestyle, the best environmental conditions possible, and adequate healthcare; and, of course, there are also a range of fundamental prerequisites for health: 'Without peace and social justice, without enough food and water, without education and decent housing, and without providing each and all with a useful role in society and an adequate income, there can be no health for the people, no real growth and no social development' (WHO, 1985).

What disabled people need, in terms of health, is much the same as anybody else. But do disabled people have access to these prerequisites for health? For example, do disabled people have access to adequate education and decent housing? And if not (because the answer is certainly no), why not?

Disability has traditionally been seen as an area of activity for medical, charitable and welfare professionals, who 'see to' disabled people on behalf of society. Disabled people have traditionally been seen as 'other' and stigmatized, even among themselves, and have been viewed as an unfortunate group of people, to be looked after by the more fortunate in society. Wielding almost absolute power over the lives of many disabled people, the charitable and 'caring' institutions and initiatives have done little, if anything, over the years to address the social exclusion we experience. Rather, they have contributed to this exclusion by segregating and marginalizing disabled people, providing 'special' schools and segregated workshops – often funded by the state – so that disabled people are stigmatized and not seen as a part of mainstream society.

In the 1970s equal opportunities legislation, in the form of the Race Relations Act and the Sex Discrimination Act, finally recognized and outlawed the discrimination experienced by many. It is only in the last five to ten years that disability has been pushed up the civil rights agenda and the issues of discrimination, segregation and oppression are beginning to take precedence over dependency, caring and curing (Davis, 1993; Driedger, 1989). This has happened almost entirely through disabled people's own efforts, through our self-organization and analysis of how society builds and maintains barriers against our participation. As an illustration, the Direct Payments Act 1996, which permits local authorities to give money direct to disabled people to buy in personal support rather than rely on inflexible local authority provision, came about entirely through lobbying by organizations controlled by disabled people.

Disabled people themselves have developed an analytical framework, the social model of disability, which notes that the exclusion experienced by disabled people comes from the barriers which society erects, and which prevent disabled people from participating in everyday activities. In the disabled people's movement we have adopted the words 'impairment' and 'disability' to describe ourselves and our situation; it is important to understand the difference between these two words. The following definition is from the British Council of Organisations of Disabled People (now British Council of Disabled People) in 1981:

> Impairment: the functional limitation within the individual caused by physical, mental or sensory impairment.
> Disability: the loss or limitations of opportunities to take part in the normal life of the community on an equal level with others due to physical and social barriers. (Barnes, 1991)

This is in contrast to the 'medical model' of disability in which the individual has something 'wrong' with them (e.g. they cannot hear) and because of that they are unable to carry out a whole range of activities, such as holding a conversation or using the telephone. This approach implies that if we cure the impairment, or seek to manage it so that people can better compete with those without impairments, then disabled people can better fit into society. This means that 'policy responses to the disadvantage experienced by disabled people have been largely concerned with individual "care", medical "cures", rehabilitation, loss adjustment, counselling, and so on' (Priestley, 1999) (see Table 4.2.1).

Location	Perceived Problem	Likely Response
Individual	misfortune	charity
	impairment	medical treatment
	otherness	segregation
	loss	adjustment
	limitation	remedial therapy
	welfare	care
Social	prejudice	public education
	poverty	disability income
	physical barriers	access
	discrimination	civil rights
	oppression	political struggle

Table 4.2.1 Policy responses to individual and social model values

The social model, however, implies that although all people are different, society does not take account of everybody's differences; if all children learnt British Sign Language at primary school, then deaf people would not need to lip-read and use interpreters. If the existing technology which produces text telephones were incorporated into our everyday phone systems, then deaf people would have access to this form of communication. The conclusion is that if we adopt a policy approach to remove the barriers to full participation (i.e. disabling attitudes, disabling environments, disabling political and economic and social structures), people would no longer be disabled but would be enabled to be active and valued members of a society that is radically altered because it embraces the diversity we bring.

The third target in support of the European regional strategy for health for all is 'Better Opportunities for the Disabled', which says: 'By the year 2000, disabled persons should have the physical, social and economic opportunities that allow at least for a socially and economically and mentally creative life' (WHO, 1985). It goes on to outline the need for programmes to develop daily living skills, easy access brought about by planning codes, improved technical aids, suitable housing, transport, paid occupations, and a guarantee of 'all the basic human rights, including the right to self determination in their own lives, to a reasonable degree of privacy, to sexual relations, and to participation in community life' (ibid.).

The civil rights agenda for disabled people in the UK peaked with the Disability Discrimination Act 1995 and the establishment in 2000 of a Disability Rights Commission. Now the disabled community holds its breath, wondering if it really will make a difference.

What can this context mean for policy and practice in public health? While public health, as a discipline, has championed and promoted measures and approaches which have impacted widely and positively on people's health, it must question whether or not it has done the same for disabled people. Policy-makers and practitioners at all levels must first look inwards to examine their own practice, and that of their colleagues and the institutions within which they work, and then look outwards at the external context, so as to influence those factors which impact negatively on the health of disabled people.

LOOKING INWARDS

Almost without exception, services which are perceived as 'mainstream' – that is, for the general population – exclude disabled people. Services which are directly health related, such as antenatal care or GP surgeries, will be designed and delivered in such a way that they do not take account of the needs of disabled people, who might instead be offered 'special' services. 'If the reality of the life experience of disabled people is to inform seriously the development of new support systems then it will be necessary to create these outside a caring paradigm which classifies all interventions in relation to disabled people within a culture of "special" needs' (Finkelstein and Stuart, 1996). Simple matters such as accessible toilets, availability of sign language interpreters, or information accessible to blind people are rarely addressed. These limitations also apply to services which, while not direct health care, contribute to the health and well-being of society – housing, education, transport, leisure, and so on.

For disabled people, access to existing services is restricted not by impairment but by barriers, whether physical, organizational, operational, or attitudinal. These barriers are installed and maintained by policy-makers and practitioners who see only the medical model of disability, and fail to take account of the needs of people with impairments. Consequently they offer services which exclude, and are often hostile to, disabled people. In addition, the experience of disability is compounded, for many people, by racism, sexism, or other forms of discrimination. Services for disabled women, for example, which are culturally sensitive are rare. As Carol Thomas points out, 'social oppressions intersect in ways which we are only beginning to explore' (1999).

LOOKING OUTWARDS

Disabled people experience disproportionate levels of poverty. Almost half (41 per cent) of economically inactive people are disabled, of whom a third (over 1 million people) would like to work (Office for National Statistics, 1999). Disabled people cannot be guaranteed a mainstream education (the Disability Discrimination Act does not yet cover education) and they do not gain access to training at the same levels as non-disabled people. Unemployment among disabled people is over twice as high as for non-disabled people: 46 per cent of disabled people are in employment, as opposed to 80 per cent of non-disabled people (Office for National Statistics, 1999). In addition, disabled people tend to be less well-qualified than their non-disabled counterparts and are more likely to work in low-skilled occupations (Department for Education and Employment, 1998).

For many disabled people, any form of public transport is inaccessible and freedom in choice of housing is rare, with some forced into residential accommodation against their will. Too often access to public spaces and buildings is a lottery. As a group, disabled people arguably experience the highest levels of social exclusion in the UK. Curiously, this is often overlooked by planners and politicians, for example, a consultation framework on the government's National Strategy for Neighbourhood Renewal, published by the Social Exclusion Unit in 2000, failed to address the existence of disabled people at all.

Public health workers and professionals are in a position, through partnerships and joint working, to promote healthy public policy across a wide constituency. All public health programmes, policies and activities, if they are to be successful, must be inclusive and must address the barriers which exclude disabled people. However, many public health promoters approach the issue of disability from the traditional medical, welfare or charitable viewpoint. Many are unaware of the social model of disability. Their activities and deliberations centre on the disabled person as 'the problem', rather than their own buildings, policies, and practices.

There are some cases where disabled people have had a positive impact on thinking and action. For example, Liverpool's Department of Public Health adopted the social model of disability in its annual report, making a commitment to work in a way that tackles the barriers to inclusion and independence. Local Agenda 21 in Manchester adopted 'access to public buildings' as a sustainability indicator. A consultancy called Equal Ability produced *Disabling Practice*, a booklet which advises on how to work better with disabled people (Equal Ability, 1999). At an organizational level, the British School of Shiatsu commissioned disability equality training through contact with a politicized deaf woman. This resulted in attitudinal changes, a close look at accommodation and in the case of one school, a move to more accessible premises and close examination of admissions procedures for students who may have additional requirements.

Good consultation pays dividends. One key issue is access to public transport, for disabled people too often an idealistic dream. However, when the Metrolink tram system in Manchester was being planned, there was informed and sustained input from disabled people into the planning and development of the trams and the infrastructure, resulting in a very accessible system. Many people remain genuinely unaware of disability matters and current thinking: disabled people's organizations offer training in disability issues, often tailored to particular situations, while some support their training with action planning sessions. Professionals and institutions need to actively seek such training, and should expect to pay a reasonable rate.

The examples above show how change can be initiated at policy and strategic levels, and also at a grass-roots service delivery level. Key to any change is an analysis of how public health workers and professionals at all levels can challenge disabling barriers. Professionals must examine their own practice and support disabled people to lead self-determined healthy lifestyles, as well as support them to tackle the barriers maintained by policies and procedures. The wider issues which public health might address, such as the impact of poverty or racism on health, or challenging negative media treatment of issues, should always include a dimension relating to disability.

Impairment need not be compounded further by imposed disability. Mainstreaming disabled people, while still accounting for their specific needs, must be the goal of inclusive public health work. Public health professionals could adopt a proactive stance by deciding to influence strategic activities and develop their own inclusive practice. This will require seeking expert advice from disabled people's own organizations on what being inclusive really means – from providing documents in pictorial format for people with learning difficulties, to ensuring facilities for guide dogs to urinate! When undertaking consultation on policies or service developments, or working 'out in the field' on health-related activities, the views of disabled people and their organizations are essential. Resources must be identified – time and support (transport to meetings or documents on tape, for example) are key to ensuring disabled people's input and, most importantly, their views must be valued. The scope for public health practitioners to be allies of the disabled people's movement is enormous, but depends on a personal and professional commitment to learn about and engage with the issues, and the people.

4.3

WOMEN AND PUBLIC HEALTH

Sue Laughlin

The language and action associated with health inequalities and social exclusion have tended largely to be dominated by concerns with socio-economic disadvantage. Other forms of inequality and discrimination that affect population groups directly, or that interact with the experience of material disadvantage, have been pushed to the margins. This has had significant implications for the development of strategic approaches aimed at promoting the health of women from the perspective of a social model of health, in which the inequality imposed by gender roles is recognized to be as important as women's reproductive systems in determining health and well-being.

This case study outlines the historical development of work in Glasgow where, despite the prevailing orthodoxy on health and considerable resistance to highlighting women's issues, a strategy for women's health has been established. It will highlight some of the achievements and some of the limitations of this work, and will consider factors which make it potentially replicable.

In 1983 a group of women working in the health authority, the local authority and a few voluntary organizations came together with community activists to organize a health event for women. The event explored a number of issues important in women's lives – employment and unemployment, women's social role, food and exercise, family life – and the likely implications for their health. A well-woman service was provided, which was particularly well received by women in their forties and older. The event attracted 6,000 women from a wide geographical area, demonstrating the demand by women to meet and consider their health in the broadest context (Greater Glasgow Health Board, 1994). It was followed up by numerous smaller events in local communities and started a dialogue between women professionals and women users of services in the city.

Subsequently, different groups of women coalesced around a campaign to extend the meaning of women's health (which led to a Women's Health Charter), and to reconfigure the nature of health provision for women. The campaign lasted for a number of years and, although there were many frustrations for those involved and in the end difficulty in sustaining commitment, there were two enduring outcomes. First, the campaign helped to consolidate an emerging analysis of women's health which, since the time of the first event, had broadened beyond the dominant medical model. Second, a Centre for Women's Health was established in 1993, funded by the health authority and regional and district local authorities.

At the same time as this activity to address women's health concerns, a more prominent transition was underway in Glasgow as the city began its involvement with the Healthy City movement. This enabled the work to raise the profile of women's health, operating mostly informally, to gain more formal recognition by becoming part of the Glasgow Healthy Cities Project, and facilitated a multi-agency group with representation from up to 50 groups and organizations (the Women's Health Working Group) in bringing forward a women's health policy for Glasgow which reflected the discussions and debates of the previous decade (Women's Health Working Group, 1996a). Launched in 1992, after a comprehensive consultation, the policy was adopted by the project partners – the health authority, the two local authorities and the University of Glasgow. A second phase of the policy was launched in 1996 to make explicit some of the concerns raised by different groups such as disabled women, and was followed by a resource manual to help organizations introduce a women's health policy at a local level (Women's Health Working Group, 1996b).

The policy was based on three underlying assumptions about the key determinants of poor health in women: women's complex reproductive system, sex and gender differences in the aetiology, diagnosis and treatment of disease, and the experience of gender inequality in society. The emphasis of the policy was to encourage organizational change, rather than focus on women's health behaviour. This is clear in the four objectives of the 1996 version of the policy:

- to increase awareness and understanding of the factors which affect the health and well-being of all women in Glasgow;
- to shape general policy development, planning and service delivery to improve the health and well-being of women;
- to ensure structures within organizations which take account of the factors which affect the health and well-being of women;
- to ensure that the key issues identified by women – which include poverty, the physical and social environment, mental health, women as carers, the needs of black and ethnic minority women, disabled women and lesbians – are addressed as priorities.

Implementation of the policy has varied across the partners of the Healthy City Project according to the extent to which there is a formal recognition of health as part of their core business. Not surprisingly, it has been easier to carry forward within Greater Glasgow Health Board and its associated NHS trusts (Laughlin, 1998), recently leading to specific commitments in the Health Improvement Programme on both women's health and gender based-violence (Greater Glasgow Health Board, 2000). Following local government reorganization in 1996, the creation of a single-tier local authority structure in Scotland appeared to weaken the political commitment to both health and women's issues in Glasgow, although the new city council remains a partner in the Healthy City Project. Although developments within the health service should be seen as positive, this has arguably distorted both the process and progress of change.

Overall, progress in implementing the policy falls into six main categories: (1) establishing organizational structures by Healthy City partners with responsibility for facilitating implementation of the policy; (2) making some services (particularly pre-existing community health services for women, and sport and leisure facilities) more women-sensitive; (3) producing and disseminating information and resources for women and about women's health (Hair, 1994; Greater Glasgow Health Board, Health Promotion Dept., 1999); (4) making and consolidating links with communities and groups of women; (5) establishing and funding a model project, the Centre for Women's Health; and (6) tackling violence against women. All these areas of progress remain under constant threat and require considerable effort to maintain at an effective level. While the overall profile of the policy – or at least some of its issues, notably violence against women – is relatively high among the city's planners and policy-makers, there has been little systematic introduction of any gender perspective into key policy areas which influence life in the city and which could have a considerable impact on health and well-being. Practical outcomes, such as the Centre for Women's Health, also remain funded outside the mainstream on a year-by-year basis.

Both the policy and the way of working in Glasgow have been adopted by the World Health Organisation as models for Europe (see Box 4.3.1) although WHO has yet to find a way of introducing such a strategic approach systematically across the Region. Similarly, there has been a virtual absence of parallel, strategic activity in other parts of the UK despite the interest of women in their health and the large number of women's health groups and projects.

BOX 4.3.1   THE GLASGOW MODEL OF WOMEN'S HEALTH

Investing in women's health

Investing in women will not only have a positive effect for women but for the population as a whole, through a reduction in inequality. There is a need to make women's health a priority because of the effects of disadvantage and discrimination that women experience.

Social model of health

This highlights the need to take a view of women's health which recognizes its social, economic and environmental determinants. It seeks to emphasize the significance of women's poverty on health. This view of health allows for the biological factors (including women's reproductive functions) which affect women, but places them in a broader framework.

A social model of health also helps to show that women are not all the same and highlights inequalities which exist between different groups of women. The Glasgow model therefore emphasizes the need to examine the specific needs, where they exist, of black and ethnic minority women, disabled women and lesbians, and develop appropriate responses.

Consultation and participation

Women have limited access to decision-making and may have limited opportunities to define their health needs. There is a need therefore to develop and implement processes which allow women to actively determine the agenda for promoting their health. (The Glasgow experience indicates that women consistently identify the promotion of emotional and mental health as their main priority.)

Inter-agency and organizational development

Liaison and co-operation with a range of organizations willing to take the lead in implementing policy are very useful. This is a prerequisite for the effective planning and delivery of all services which have an impact on health.

Strategic framework

It follows from the above that a strategic framework with the following elements is required which would incorporate:

- women's community development to help articulate health concerns;
- an intersectoral forum for women's health which brings together statutory organizations, voluntary organizations and community groups to identify priorities;
- women's health policy development and implementation;
- organizational structures and systems which raise awareness and facilitate data collection by gender, gender monitoring and gender-sensitive planning;
- a centre for women's health to try out new methods of responding effectively to women's unmet health needs;
- research and development of indicators of women's well-being.

In many ways, then, the work in Glasgow can be considered an anachronism, struggling as it has against two major ideological difficulties: the continuing dominance of the medical model in determining health policy and resource allocation, and the marginalization of feminism. The weight of these difficulties may account for the absence elsewhere of the kind of work that has taken place in Glasgow. Nonetheless, the experience has shown that even in unfavourable conditions there can be progress, and it is useful to consider the possible factors that may account for that progress and make replication elsewhere possible.

First, the work was undeniably aided by the presence of advocates with sufficient status to have some influence in both the health and local authorities and the persistence to try to promote a women's agenda. Second, the struggle for change combined, for much of the period described, action within organizations and pressure from women's groups outside, much of it co-ordinated through the Clydeside Women's Health Campaign. A third factor was the conceptual origins and ongoing perspective of women's health, which had more in common with the 'new public health', albeit from a feminist perspective, than with the traditional interests of the women's health movement in women's rights within the medical system and the demedicalization of women's reproductive health problems.

A fourth consideration was the development of a strategic perspective which focused on multi-agency organizational development rather than on changing the behaviour of women or individual practitioners. At the same time, a dialogue between some policy-makers and practitioners and women and women's groups informed the changes sought, although the differences in power and status between these groups inevitably meant the dialogue was imperfect.

The demonstration project, the Centre for Women's Health, played a key role in that it sought to integrate service provision with a strategic function which attempted to inform mainstream service delivery to respond more effectively to women's health needs.

The final factor was the local and national struggle for public recognition of the abuse of women by men. Until recently this struggle co-existed with the work on women's health more generally but there has been a gradual convergence over recent years as the poor health associated with violence has become more apparent (Scottish Needs Assessment Programme, 1997), helping to highlight the link between women's health and the experience of gender inequality.

It is worth noting the general environment in which the work in Glasgow has been operating. Unlike some other countries – Australia or Canada, for example – there has been no national policy for promoting the health of women which properly recognizes its social context. Undoubtedly, this can partly be attributed to inherent sexism within government departments, despite their sporadic attempts to raise the profile of women's health (Department of Health, 1996) and the new interest in gender mainstreaming (MacKay and Bilton, 2000).

But perhaps more significantly, the movements which have been pressing for a 'new public health' perspective have been similarly gender blind and this can also be considered a form of institutional sexism. Although there has been recent progress in recognizing health inequalities, as a result of lobbying from the public health movement, this has focused primarily on socio-economic inequalities in health. As long as this remains the sole emphasis, developing a strategic approach to women's health which recognizes its social and economic determinants will remain difficult.

Societies have been described as being divided along the 'fault-line' of gender (Doyal, 1995). Women and men have different health needs which stem partly from biological differences and partly from their relative social positions. Until acting on this understanding becomes a priority for those concerned with equity in health and health care, there are limits to how the health of many women – and men – may be improved. The new public health/health promotion movements must respond to this challenge first, by acknowledging the significance of gender as a determinant of health; second, by recognizing the adverse health impact of sex discrimination; and third, by devoting as much energy to lobbying on these issues as that previously expended on the health effects of poverty.

5

REGENERATION AND HEALTH

Hilary Russell

Health to me is about decent housing, nice neighbours, good friends, not feeling isolated, having enough money to live on, having a clean environment, and some community facilities and resources. (A 50-year-old single mother quoted in Dunne, 1993)

This chapter looks at the relationship between regeneration and health. A brief review of changing approaches to both health and regeneration illustrates the importance of conceptual definitions and understandings in shaping policies, even though the underpinning assumptions of policy were sometimes demonstrably wrong. During the 1990s, a more comprehensive approach to regeneration brought recognition of its potential health impacts and started to include specific 'health' projects. The current policy climate provides opportunities for a more strategic approach. Lessons from the past can usefully inform how these opportunities are grasped. Early experiences of strategic working suggest challenges and tensions but also the potential for greater long term effectiveness.

CHANGING EMPHASES IN HEALTH POLICY

Policy thinking on health has seen various swings of the pendulum. There is an argument that urban policy in its widest sense originated with the public health tradition and its attempts to control the environmental causes of disease (Blackman, 1995). It became very evident in the nineteenth century that the urban environment – homes, neighbourhoods and workplaces – had a significant effect upon people's health. Associated with this recognition came increased attention to collecting and analysing epidemiological data. Reforms were sought through legislation and improved standards in housing, sanitation and workplace safety, interventions specifically acknowledging the need to prevent ill-health by addressing non-health factors which were determinants of health.

Divergence between evidence and policy

However, by the middle of the twentieth century, it was assumed that the welfare state made sufficient provision for people's basic needs. Emphasis switched, therefore, to achieving medical advances and improving standards of health care. But inequalities in health persisted across social class divisions and across areas in terms of mortality, morbidity, accidents and the use of health services. Although The Black Report acknowledged there was no single, simple explanation for the complex data assembled, it did stress the importance of material conditions: 'In our view much of the evidence on social inequalities in health can be adequately understood in terms of specific features of the socio-economic environment' (Townsend and Davidson, 1982). The report also suggested an 'area deprivation' strategy, on the lines of Educational Priority Areas or Housing Action Areas, targeted on the ten authorities with the highest death rates. But the Conservative government at the time preferred to attribute primary responsibility for ill health to individual lifestyle choices (Jones, 1997). It disputed the working party's findings and rejected its recommendations. Later, even though *Health of the Nation* (Department of Health, 1992) high-lighted disease prevention and health education, it continued to emphasize educating individuals and persuading them to adopt healthier lifestyles. While government underlined the importance of biomedical risk factors, it discounted other risk conditions such as poverty or unemployment as well as psychosocial factors such as social isolation, low self-esteem and powerlessness (Labonte, 1995).

Despite continuing evidence supporting a holistic model of health and demonstrating the relevance of physical, emotional, psychological, social and intellectual factors (the 'Pepsi' concept, Calman, 1998: 5), few explicit connections were made between health and regeneration initiatives through the 1980s and early 1990s. Before turning to the increasing convergence between the two agendas that has occurred since the mid-1990s, it is worth looking at the evolution of regeneration policy.

THREE DECADES OF URBAN POLICY

For most of the past 30 years, regeneration has been largely synonymous with urban regeneration. British urban policy has deployed multiple policy initiatives and instruments, changing as political priorities and views about the nature of urban problems changed. They variously targeted particular social groups or areas, identified individual or structural causes, responded to social need or economic opportunity, focused upon social support or economic development. Different players or sectors occupied the driving seat at different times. The trigger for the introduction of urban policy in the 1960s was the persistence of urban poverty despite the welfare state. This, combined with anxiety about race relations, prompted the creation of the Urban Programme. The Programme's scope and management reflected the diagnosis of the problems on which it was based. It had limited resources and was project-led.

> It assumed inner city problems were caused by the individual failings of a limited number of people who lacked the skills to succeed economically. In other words, it blamed the victim. The programme was managed by the Home Office precisely because it was responsible for police and immigration.

The urban problem was ghettoised in more than one sense as government commitment to the cities was tentative at best. (Parkinson, 1995)

The early establishment of 12 Community Development Projects (CDPs), exposed the inadequacy of this approach. Research emerging from them underlined the need to address the structural economic causes of inner-city problems rather than focus only on their social consequences. The 1977 White Paper, *The Inner Cities*, 'which has yet to be bettered in terms of analysis or prescription' (Parkinson, 1995) ushered in a shift in Labour government policy based on a different understanding of urban change and setting aside the 'pathological view' of inner-city problems. Larger main programme budgets were to be bent in favour of cities with the increased, though still modest, Urban Programme funds acting as a 'sweetener' to bring in other players. Management of the Urban Programme now switched to the Department of the Environment. 'Inner City Partnerships' were created in the six largest cities, prefiguring many of the values, ambitions and priorities of initiatives in the 1990s. In particular, they sought to combine economic, social and environmental regeneration. They failed partly because of policy design weaknesses, but perhaps more significantly because the incoming Conservative government in 1979 redefined the 'inner city problem' yet again (Robson, 1988), went off in a new policy direction and cut funding for the partnerships.

Urban entrepreneurialism

In the 1980s, economic and physical regeneration led by the private sector was seen as the key to the revival of the inner cities. The government saw market failure as the key problem behind the flight of investment and physical decline, and market forces as the solution. 'The engine of enterprise was now the driving force of inner city policies' (Deakin and Edwards, 1993). 'Wealth creation' was narrowly defined and equated with the private sector, with public sector organizations often seen as impeding the effective operation of the free market. The government's ideological hostility towards the welfare state in the 1980s was manifest in a deliberate move away from redistributive welfare and fiscal policies. Instead, the assumption was that 'a rising tide would lift all ships' – that is, economic growth would raise overall standards. However, as free market mechanisms notoriously produce winners and losers, it was in practice a 'strategy of inequality' (Walker, 1990).

By the end of the 1980s, although the first wave of Urban Development Corporations may have fulfilled their brief in the strict sense of producing new infrastructure, their achievements were geographically and socially restricted. They had little impact on adjacent communities in terms of environmental improvements, housing, jobs or training. Later, some attempted to redress the balance (Russell, 1998), but the impression lingered that local people bore many of the costs of this type of regeneration while gaining few of the benefits.

A large-scale study (Robson et al., 1994) examining the package of Action for Cities policy instruments introduced in the 1980s came to mixed conclusions about their impact. Although many urban areas saw some relative improvement, the seven largest cities experienced both relative and absolute decline and the problems of their most deprived areas had seeped out more generally. The question remained whether they would have fared even less well without the various urban initiatives. Despite this, the experience of the 1980s underlined the crucial importance of the whole range of public policy in shaping quality of life: both directly through its effect on the country's economic and social structure and indirectly through the parameters set for local action.

Towards a comprehensive approach to regeneration

> It is clear, then, that the inner cities – or parts of them – have not shared the benefits of rapid economic growth. Why is this so? Why, if there are available resources in terms of labour and land, has the 'invisible hand' not reached further into these pockets of urban deprivation? (Audit Commission, 1989: 12)

Harrison wrote: 'The state of the inner city in the early 1980s is . . . a warning of what much of Britain's urban future may look like unless there is a radical change in policies' (1983: 25). What he saw were events and processes that were not new but had been brought to a head by the combined pressures of global recession and monetarist policies. Not just a symptom and a warning, the inner city was also a symbol. 'It is the place where all our social ills come together, the place where all our sins are paid for' (ibid.: 21). The term 'inner city' was more than a label for defined areas. It signified a quality of urban problems which may have been found in inner cities but also characterized some outer estates and parts of small towns. By the end of the 1980s, this spatial pattern of decline was irrefutable. The new policy direction of the 1990s was partly driven by growing realization that the 'trickle down' theory of economic growth did not work. Poverty and unemployment were not just features of an economy in recession. They were equally by-products of booming economies. Unchecked market forces led to accelerating polarization and the marginalization of the most vulnerable groups and areas. Two-speed cities were developing. Economic competitiveness was being bought at the cost of social cohesion.

Recognition of the multi-dimensional and interrelated character of deprivation led to more holistic area-based regeneration, with an emphasis on partnerships between agencies. Initiatives such as City Challenge, the Single Regeneration Budget Challenge Fund (SRB) and, in Scotland, the Programme for Partnerships, incorporated past lessons, in principle, even if only falteringly in practice:

- the value of public, private, voluntary and community sector partnerships;
- the need for local authorities to have greater powers and resources;
- the need for greater governmental co-ordination;
- the need to target the benefits of regeneration on disadvantaged groups.

City Challenge, and later SRB, hinged upon a concept of partnership that was fundamental to achieving strategic consistency and collaboration, and maximizing the effective use of resources. Greater recognition of the interrelationships between social and economic factors led to new programmes, giving greater scope for social regeneration. Beginning particularly with City Challenge, initiatives increasingly incorporated health in their programmes. The trend was further encouraged by growing attention to community consultation and involvement. Lay definitions of health tend to echo the breadth of the holistic model and cover both the negative aspects of disease and impaired function and the positive ones of well-being and enhanced function (Blaxter, 1990). Once local people were asked about their concerns, not only did issues such as health and community safety assume much greater prominence, but the connections began to be made with wider socio-economic conditions.

MAKING THE LINKS BETWEEN REGENERATION AND HEALTH

In the late 1980s and early 1990s, the concept of social exclusion started to become more widespread in the European Union. Initially a backdoor way of talking about poverty when some EU member state governments were disinclined to admit its existence, social exclusion has become a much broader concept. More dynamic, relational and multi-dimensional, it signifies a process as much as a condition. It turns the focus onto the structural roots of poverty, not just its personal consequences. It involves labour markets, housing markets, welfare systems and many other facets of the economic and social order that contribute to or detract from quality of life. Provided that it does not obscure the still fundamental importance of income, this understanding is a more constructive basis for formulating policy.

CUMULATIVE AND INTERCONNECTED PROBLEMS

Localities targeted in area-based regeneration, whatever their other differences, have tended to share a range of problems and socio-economic characteristics. Compared with national, regional and sub-regional averages, they typically have more households receiving income support, more pupils eligible for free school meals, high levels of unemployment and long-term unemployment, degraded housing stock and higher recorded crime rates. Health problems are reflected in higher infant mortality rates, higher proportions of underweight births, higher perinatal mortality and higher standardized mortality rates (Russell et al., 1996; SEU, 1998).

Regeneration initiatives themselves, especially where they successfully involve local people, have served to increase awareness of the interconnected and cumulative nature of these dimensions of social exclusion, including its health impacts:

- low-income levels are often associated with poor diet and heating;
- poverty and debt lead to anxiety, feelings of inadequacy and a breakdown in family relationships;
- unemployment can impair mental and physical health;

- homelessness and poor housing have effects ranging from increased mental health problems to a higher rate of accidents in the home, respiratory illnesses, and a lower level of resistance to disease;
- the multiple effects of social exclusion exacerbate other problems, isolate people and erode social ties;
- areas of concentrated deprivation frequently have poorer facilities and services, including health care;
- deprived areas may have higher levels of crime and fear of crime, which promote feelings of insecurity and change behaviour in ways that restrict choices and quality of life;
- conversely, lower standards of health depress productivity and increase social and financial costs.

Although these connections had long been recognized by some and were embodied in projects such as Healthy Cities, they had been little acknowledged by governments.

TACKLING THE RANGE OF ISSUES AFFECTING HEALTH

The mix of economic and social goals in the comprehensive approach to regeneration resulted in a wide range of activities. Table 5.1 gives examples under four headings:

- economic development, focusing on demand side issues, aiming to increase and diversify economic activity;
- employment, training and education dealing with supply side issues and obstacles to people entering the labour market;
- improving housing and the residential environment by producing better and more appropriate physical stock, creating safer neighbourhoods and involving residents in managing their neighbourhoods;
- quality of life strategies including attention to health but also extending to policy areas such as community development, leisure and community safety.

Such activities variously connect with each 'layer' of the main determinants of health: general socio-economic, cultural and environmental conditions; living and working conditions; social and community influences; and individual lifestyle factors (Dahlgren and Whitehead, 1991). They also span the four main levels of policy response: strengthening individuals; strengthening communities; improving access to essential facilities and services; and encouraging macroeconomic and cultural change (Whitehead, 1995).

DIVERSE APPROACHES

Many projects have explicitly or implicitly recognized the links between social and economic conditions and physical, mental and emotional health. Some responses represent 'coping' strategies: for example, enabling people to make a

Economic development – enterprise support	Employment, training, education
land reclamation	practical help to employers with
provision of new industrial and	recruitment and training
office space	job link schemes
infrastructural improvements	local labour co-ordinators for
environmental improvements	construction work
in industrial areas	provision of affordable childcare
CCTV and other security measures	customized pre-recruitment training
provision of venture capital	packages
industrial grants	skills audits and registers
business loan funds	guidance for job applicants on job
mentoring schemes	hunting, benefits, training and careers
local purchasing/inter-trading schemes	pre-vocational training – access and
one-stop shops	basic skills
	customized training
	access courses for HE
	curriculum support projects
	out-of-school learning projects
	capital schemes to improve school
	facilities
	development workers in schools
	anti-bullying and anti-racist projects
Housing and residential environment	**Quality of life**
estate remodelling	grants and support to voluntary and
environmental improvement	community groups
traffic calming	planning for real exercises
demolition and new build	improvement of play areas and
self-build schemes	facilities
provision for special needs groups	new community centres
including foyer schemes	community safety measures
security improvements and security grants	diversionary schemes as alternatives
CCTV	to crime for young people
energy efficiency schemes	health houses and health groups
tenant management initiatives	health studies – e.g. epidemiology; air
	quality
	arts and cultural projects
	improvement of leisure and social
	facilities

Table 5.1
Examples of
activities directed
towards economic
and social goals

Source: Russell et al., 1996

low income stretch further through food co-operatives or classes in low budget cookery (LGA, 1998a). Other approaches have been preventative: for example, raising income levels, enabling people to access employment and taking steps to improve housing. Increasing awareness of the need to promote more stable and sustainable communities (Page, 1994; Thake, 1995; Gowman, 1999) is only partly a matter of the physical environment (Urban Task Force, 1999). It extends to strengthening social ties through a balanced social mix, the necessary social infrastructure, accessible services, and fostering resident involvement. There is a strong link between general satisfaction with a neighbourhood and perceptions of its friendliness (Ambrose, 1996).

Recent policy development has stressed not just policy goals but the processes of promoting change. Despite varying views about the nature of community life, many commentators regard the community as an important level of intervention. Community-based regeneration, harnessing the strengths of community groups, focuses upon developing social businesses and other activities, such as credit unions, community co-operatives and local exchange trading schemes (LETS), which develop and consolidate local micro-economies. Increasing the circulation of money within, and halting its flow out of, an area is important to a community's self-reliance and social cohesion.

The neighbourhood, as much as the individual, must be the focus of health promotion (Gillies, 1998). Influences on health include social support, social networks and social roles and activities. Deprivation can have a negative effect on health by undermining the health-enhancing stocks of social capital (Gillies et al., 1996). Although the concept of social capital remains elusive and disputed, in time it may help to explain how community factors affect health and provide criteria for interventions beneficial to health.

PIECEMEAL TO INTEGRATED

We believe in working across Government to attack the breeding ground of poor health – poverty and social exclusion – and we believe in creating strong local partnerships with local authorities, health authorities and other agencies to tackle the root causes of ill-health in places where people live. (Department of Health (DH), 1999b: 3)

A new agenda

Acknowledging the range of policy areas that impact on health and the importance of process issues were important steps forward. However, piecemeal and project-based initiatives alone cannot make a long-term impact on health inequalities (Russell with Killoran, 2000). The Labour government in 1997 heralded a new agenda for health and regeneration. A greater concern with addressing need was signalled both by the appointment of the first-ever Minister for Public Health and by the creation of the Social Exclusion Unit with the remit to improve government action to promote social inclusion by producing 'joined up solutions to joined up problems'. The change of direction was especially pronounced in health with the introduction of Health Improvement Programmes, Health Action Zones and Healthy Living Centres in the health green and white papers (DH 1997; 1998; 1999b) and the early commissioning of a review of health inequalities (Acheson, 1998). In addition, stronger emphasis on equity and on adopting an approach based on the twin principles of partnership and community involvement have brought health and regeneration initiatives much closer together. Both face similar challenges. Nationally and locally, it is necessary to do the following:

- find the right spatial level of intervention;
- ensure that national, regional and local policies interact effectively;
- achieve effective co-ordination between different parts of government, different agencies and different sectors.

A review of lessons from regeneration initiatives to date (DETR, 1997) identified themes also clearly applicable to health regarding:

- strategic and holistic approaches;
- mainstreaming the approach;
- being outcome-focused in planning strategies and front line operations;
- marrying ameliorative and preventative activity;
- targeting and concentrating resources to avoid diluting their impact;
- finding new forms of strategic and operational partnership;
- achieving a whole systems approach to institutional change across disciplinary, professional and agency boundaries;
- involving and building the capacity of local communities;
- finding new ways of working and of defining and measuring success.

Strategic opportunities

Health Action Zones (HAZs) and New Commitment to Regeneration (NCR) provide the opportunity to apply these lessons. HAZs were established to act as 'a framework for the NHS, local authorities and other partners to work together to achieve progress in addressing the causes of ill-health and reducing health inequalities' (Department of Health, 1998). HAZ status was given for seven years. The first HAZs were established as pilot schemes in November 1998 and the second wave became effective from April 1999. They have two strategic objectives: to identify and address the public health needs of the local area, in particular piloting new ways of tackling health inequalities; and to modernize services by increasing their effectiveness, efficiency and responsiveness.

NCR is a strategic approach to regeneration developed by the Local Government Association in partnership with a range of national and local organizations and with government support. Applicable in urban and rural areas, it draws on past lessons (Wilks-Heeg, 2000) and differs from previous regeneration initiatives in involving:

- whole local authority areas or combinations of local authorities;
- the mainstream programmes and budgets of all the public agencies in an area;
- national government as a key partner;
- the exploration and development of freedoms and flexibilities in how national programmes are implemented locally.

Together these design elements provide the basis for going beyond a 'hot spots' approach to regeneration. While revitalizing poor neighbourhoods remains a high priority for government, it also concedes that past failure resulted from the lack of a coherent strategy and that, too often, there has been a confusion of responsibilities between area-based regeneration schemes and core public services (SEU, 2000b). Area-based regeneration has often been limited because the necessary changes were beyond the powers of local actors or needed intervention at a wider spatial level. Some policy commentators have warned against over-reliance upon area-based schemes (Townsend, 1991). Although they have an important supplementary role, they should not distract from the significance of the national management of the economy and accompanying social policies in influencing local economic and social conditions and creating the framework for resolving local problems.

Where there is widespread deprivation, NCR gives a framework for making regeneration – in the widest sense of sustainability – the driving rationale for managing the city, county or conurbation. Though not precluding the need to target smaller areas for improvement, it allows for a more inclusive strategy. More poor and excluded people live outside than inside deprived neighbourhoods. Some equity issues need tackling through wider interventions, mainstream programmes and the deployment of resources at a higher spatial level. NCR recognizes that deprived areas cannot be treated in isolation, but need to be seen in the context of their interrelationship with other neighbourhoods and as part of the wider economic scene. It offers the possibility of a more integrated approach to balancing social, economic and environmental goals in relation to the different problems and challenges of rural as well as urban areas.

NCR is being tested in areas designated as 'Pathfinders'. It 'directly complements many of the things the Government is trying to achieve, especially through the modernisation of local government and the emphasis on community planning; the work of the Social Exclusion Unit; and a range of area-based initiatives' (LGA, 1998b).

By early 2000, both the NCR partnerships and HAZs were being seen as potential bases for the Local Strategic Partnerships (LSPs) proposed in the SEU *National Strategy for Neighbourhood Renewal* (SEU, 2000c). The purpose of LSPs would be to bring together service providers, local organizations and residents to improve services in deprived neighbourhoods and address cross-cutting issues such as social exclusion. The same principles are echoed in the government guidance on *Preparing Community Strategies* (DETR, 2000d), which talks about community planning partnerships putting together community strategies which 'should aim to enhance the quality of life of local communities through action to improve the economic, social and environmental well-being of an area and its inhabitants'.

Delivering a new approach

The experience of NCR Pathfinders (Russell, 2000) and HAZs to date can provide early lessons about strategic partnership working. The potentially radical new approach that they bring requires a drastic redefinition of organizational values and cultures and new forms of management and delivery. As they are both underpinned by principles of partnership, staff involvement and community involvement, it is important for HAZs and NCR partnerships to do the following:

- provide a framework for connecting special, area-based and/or time-limited initiatives with the mainstream;
- achieve strategic integration: horizontally across agencies and vertically at different spatial levels with neighbourhood, regional and national policies;
- develop a strategic framework for putting partnership into practice.

Developing trust, building partnerships and establishing appropriate structures take considerable time but are essential for successful collaboration. *Equipping for partnership* depends upon an ethos of partnership within as well as between organizations extending to service users and the wider community. Real, embedded partnership working will permeate and change member organizations as well as leading to wider structures of partnership and new joint working mechanisms such as service level agreements, contracts and protocols. It may require new organizational arrangements, relationships and skills and entail new job descriptions and cross-disciplinary and cross-agency staff development. New ways of working will also call for new mechanisms for democratic accountability. However, although increased joint working will challenge traditional ways of working, partnership should also mean respecting difference and capitalizing upon the distinctive approaches and contributions of partner organizations.

Making partnership happen requires leadership and a dedicated delivery vehicle to act as a stimulus and catalyst for policy linkages, maintaining the collaborative focus and building joint capacity. Over the past decade, it has been recognized that comprehensive regeneration requires a cluster of skills (SEU, 2000b) generic to different policy areas, including partnership skills such as listening and learning from others, team building and working with communities. Strategic partnerships may similarly signal the need for a specific form of professional expertise, this time revolving around creative networking across the 'virtual community' of partner organizations. The language and skills of community development (Gilchrist, 2000) have a lot to offer in this new context towards the goal of establishing a 'well-connected community' in which 'people feel part of a web of diverse and inter-locking relationships'.

Reciprocal government action

Achieving 'joined-up responses' requires reciprocal action by national government. If local organizations are being told to come out of their 'silos', national government must also overcome compartmentalization and policy fragmentation. 'Central government is not "joined up". This is both a symbolic barrier as there is no role model for joined-up behaviour at the local level, and a practical barrier as it makes it more difficult to generate cohesion between initiatives at the local level.' Whitehall is ill-equipped for managing cross-cutting policies and services (PIU, 2000a, 2000b). The proliferation of new initiatives since 1997 has become confusing and their strong centralized direction is counter-productive.

A key feature of NCR Pathfinders is their diversity in type of area, their socio-economic and institutional contexts, their histories and traditions of partnership working, their experiences of regeneration, their strategic priorities. HAZs are similarly diverse. Local players want government to recognize this diversity and move away from the 'one size fits all' packaging of policy, allowing greater autonomy for local organizations to choose the most appropriate ways of meeting their own and national policy targets. If outcomes are the key measure of success, then it is essential to shed the national straitjacket.

Government must work out the implications of central–local partnership for its own behaviour. On the one hand, it means taking responsibility for those outcomes which can only be reached through policies implemented at national level. On the other, government must provide a more 'user-friendly' operating environment for local organizations, including more scope for joining up budgets and a performance management framework which encourages and rewards joint working.

Adding value through a strategic approach

Being outcome oriented is the central strand from which all else flows. The determinants of health do not fall neatly into the remit of any single agency or department. Improving health and well-being, therefore, demands an integrated and long term strategy. 'Joined-up thinking', 'cross-cutting', 'partnership' and 'innovation' have all become *de rigueur*. It is time to take further steps towards turning the rhetoric into reality.

5.1

THE WAKEFIELD HEALTH ACTION ZONE: A CASE STUDY IN AREA-FOCUSED WORKING

Lee Adams

Health Action Zones are part of the New Labour project to improve health, reduce inequalities and improve health services. They were announced in Labour's first White Paper on the NHS, *The New NHS – Modern, Dependable* (Department of Health, 1997), and more detail was given in the public health strategy *Our Healthier Nation* (Department of Health, 1998). A first wave of areas gained HAZ status in 1998, with a second wave following in 1999, following a competitive application process. In total, England has 26 HAZs, and Northern Ireland has two.

HAZs are diverse in both size and composition, ranging from what are effectively regional zones (for example, Tyne and Wear) to smaller areas such as the town of Luton. Some share the same boundaries as the health authority and local government authority for the area, such as Bradford. Others are more complex, including multiple authorities or part of a health authority within their area.

The zones are responsible to their local health authorities, which in turn are accountable to health ministers through the NHS Executive. At the same time, however, HAZs are supposed to be a partnership of the key agencies in a district. This creates an immediate contradiction and challenge, since in theory all partners should take equal responsibility for the HAZ, yet formal accountability remains entirely within the NHS.

HAZs are located within a government agenda of 'modernizing' the NHS. This programme includes work to restore public confidence, to integrate health and social care to provide seamless services, to promote a service that is quick to respond to urgent need, is effective, equitable, patient-centred and accessible, and in which users are involved in planning and monitoring services and their outcomes. In addition, HAZs have a remit to promote health and reduce health inequality through enabling and supporting partnerships across the public, private, non-profit and community sectors.

HAZs are different from other area initiatives in that they also have a role in promoting cultural change, co-ordinating action within an area to improve health and well-being, not just of the different sectors' work, but of area-based and other strategic initiatives. There is a tension in this, in that HAZs are also trying to develop equal and complementary partnerships with other area-based initiatives, as well as play a co-ordinating role (LGA, 2000a).

WAKEFIELD AND DISTRICT HEALTH ACTION ZONE

The Wakefield HAZ, which is coterminous with the metropolitan district council and health authority boundaries, includes Wakefield itself, five towns in the surrounding area (Pontefract, Knottingley, Castleford, Normanton and Hemsworth) and many smaller settlements. The original plan for the HAZ was developed in early 1999, based upon existing data about health, social, economic and environmental needs together with consultation responses to the Health Improvement Programme.

Some additional consultation was also undertaken, and partner agencies were involved in agreeing the plan. The HAZ partner agencies form a co-ordination group, whose members are the health authority, Wakefield Metropolitan District Council, local NHS trusts, primary care trusts, the voluntary sector and representation from trade unions, users and carers and the local Wakefield College. The co-ordination group reports to the local strategic partnership and is chaired by the council cabinet lead on health, housing and social care. The chamber of commerce and the training and enterprise council, local MPs, and nearby universities were also asked to comment on the plan, and are involved in groups which discuss the HAZ and the local health improvement plan.

In the HAZ plan we argued why the area needed HAZ status. Like other deprived areas, our district has a social and economic history that has left a legacy of poor health and inequality. The collapse of the coal mining industry devastated the area and its people, creating mass unemployment, a poor physical environment, and a widespread sense of hopelessness, with an inevitable cost in terms of physical and mental health (Wakefield HAZ, 1999; Wakefield MDC, 1998). As well as evidence of need, our plan was also based on evidence about how public health can be improved (Wakefield HAZ, 2001).

The definition of health we developed and used throughout the plan and its implementation is a social one: 'Health is a state of wellbeing. Healthy people feel good, have all their basic needs met and are able to realise their potential and relate well to others. Health is affected by many things but the most influential are social, economic and environmental' (Wakefield HAZ, 1999).

While many public health initiatives are aimed at specific diseases (a 'vertical' approach), a large amount of evidence suggests we should focus on the determinants of health, trying to ensure the basic necessities of life are available to all (a 'horizontal' approach), and this is the approach we have taken in the HAZ. Among 'basic necessities' we include good nutrition, social and emotional support, decent and warm housing, adequate income, meaningful work in a healthy workplace, healthy environments, opportunities for education and to contribute to community life, and the availability of support services.

In setting out this approach we drew on the work of national and international researchers who had documented the existing, and widening, inequalities in health; the work of Richard Wilkinson (1996) and others on material deprivation, relative poverty, exclusion and its impact upon health and quality of life; work that pointed to the need to focus on the determinants of health to reduce inequality; and theories of sustainable development (Wakefield HAZ, 2001). In terms of service change, we drew upon systematic reviews and evidence-based guidelines for good practice.

As HAZ director, I also influenced the programme from my own experience of 25 years working in public health in the NHS, my beliefs about ethical ways to work (Adams and Pintus, 1994; French and Adams, 1996) and what I knew would make a difference. Our programme was also based on the recommendations from the Acheson inquiry into health inequalities (Acheson, 1998), although we recognized the limitations of these and the scope of the work undertaken (UKPHA, 1999). Naturally, we also addressed the government agenda.

To guide the work we set out 13 principles, based on ethical and effective practice and influenced by the Ottawa Charter, the WHO Health For All programme, and the Agenda 21 strategy (UN, 1992b). In essence, the plan was shaped around five core objectives:

1 Developing community participation, capacity and supporting community development – drawing on the evidence of social capital, social support, community development and its impact upon health.
2 Promoting positive health – trying to re-orientate health and related services to a preventive, holistic and positive approach.
3 Tackling the root causes of ill health, drawing on the conclusive evidence of the importance of material conditions, social structures and environments on health.
4 Improving services and integrating and modernising provision from the user's perspective.
5 Creating a 'HAZ culture' and infrastructures locally to sustain the activity.

We set out the indicators and goals we were trying to achieve. These have now been further refined through the evaluation work (Alcock et al., 2000; 2001) and are being used to inform a set of integrated indicators for quality of life in the district (Wakefield MDC, 1999–2001).

PRACTICAL EXAMPLES FROM THE PROGRAMME

The HAZ funds around 50 specific initiatives, and in addition undertakes considerable organizational, community and cultural development and change activities. More than simply the sum of its parts, the HAZ was designed and works as a matrix, with all activities working together to the common objectives. Our plan is complex and different from some other HAZ plans, in that it focuses on many areas as opposed to a few. This was deliberate, because there was so much need and a lot of organizational and community capacity to build. A narrower approach would have satisfied very few stakeholders. We now have a rich programme with interlocking themes. Examples of the work and our achievements over the first year are given in Box 5.2.1.

BOX 5.2.1   ACHIEVEMENTS OF THE WAKEFIELD HAZ

Participation, capacity building and community development

Supporting people with disabilities to ensure their rights under the Disability Discrimination Act and to promote community development, and participation to improve services.
Building the voluntary sector, which is very under-resourced in the district, in order to develop youth volunteering and establish a volunteer bureau.
Supporting a new forum for users of mental health services.
Establishing community development and health work in several poor areas.
Supporting work to extend tenants' involvement and capacity building.

Promoting positive health

Undertaking development work with 13 emerging community-led healthy living initiatives.
Involving young people in taking action on sexual health.
Funding a healthy schools programme.
Establishing health promotion initiatives with young people, older people, and people with learning disabilities.

Tackling the root causes of ill health

Supporting many vulnerable young people, care leavers, homeless and offenders to access housing, social support, and drug programmes, and parenting programmes.
Providing vulnerable homeless people with rent deposits to secure housing.
Developing a nutrition and food poverty programme and action to create food co-ops.
Providing benefits uptake work in primary care.
Developing a credit union for Wakefield City.
Conducting an environmental health mapping for the district and developing impact assessment frameworks.

Improving health and social care services

Training 100 professionals to support smokers who want to quit, and establishing a specialist service.
Extending a cardiac rehabilitation scheme based in community care to enable it to be available to all patients that need it in the second year of HAZ.
Developing a plan for mental health which had 22 HAZ-funded initiatives in support of the objectives and standards.

Establishing fellowships in areas of anxiety management, reducing deliberate self-harm, developing creative therapy for vulnerable young people, and developing a chronic lung disease programme in primary care.

Developing two projects to provide support to young offenders who use drugs to stay off and stay clear of crime, and a programme in the local prisons to provide better care for inmates with asthma or diabetes.

Supporting the reconfiguration of health service planning to enable a whole systems approach to prevention, primary, secondary and tertiary care linked to community development and regeneration in the district.

Developing cancer care pathways.

Creating cultural change and building infrastructures

More than doubling the HAZ budget through gaining matched funding, mainly from the EU.

Working to support the community plan for the district, with policy staff of the Wakefield Metropolitan District Council.

Working closely with SRB programmes, financing the development work of Sure Start, and having joint programmes with the Education Action Zone.

Working to integrate the health improvement plan and the community plan.

Developing a joint framework for community participation, and making the case for and supporting a joint community development strategy.

Developing multi-disciplinary public health specialists.

Creating a joint interagency team – Action For Health – to help facilitate all the above, with staff with a range of skills in health development and public health, social and economic policy analysis, planning, health promotion, organization and community development, and with a wide range of backgrounds.

(Wakefield HAZ, 2000)

The HAZ has supported and developed partnership working in the district. For social, economic and environmental well-being the local strategic partnership required by government will integrate these elements (DETR, 2000a).

EVALUATION

The HAZ is being evaluated both as part of a national evaluation, undertaken by a team from Glasgow University, and through a locally commissioned evaluation led by Professor Peter Alcock of Birmingham University. Both evaluations are using a theories of change and realistic evaluation approach (Judge et al., 1999a, b). The local evaluation is working with the HAZ initiatives in defining common goals, supporting projects to self-evaluate as well as conducting an in-depth evaluation of several representative projects and an overall evaluation, using a variety of methods both quantitative and qualitative.

In the first year the local evaluation team stated:

> The major achievement of the HAZ in its early phase of operation has been to bring about a cultural change within some of the key agencies and build a willingness to work within a partnership framework . . .
> A key achievement has been to establish a partnership approach to tackling health inequalities . . .
> The HAZ has generated very real enthusiasm and provided opportunities for innovation and organisational change. (Alcock et al., 2000)

The Wakefield HAZ has been successful during its first two years. As well as the evaluation, HAZ performance is monitored through mechanisms that measure progress against objectives for each initiative. Each HAZ is also monitored by the NHS Executive, through a logical framework approach, in which each initiative is assessed in terms of progress in achieving defined goals. Although it is not possible to generalize from Wakefield, it is fair to suggest that the HAZs are very carefully monitored and evaluated.

DISCUSSION

Although there have been many achievements, there have been things that have not gone smoothly, including some under-spending of our budget in year one because it took time to develop robust projects, and organizational processes slowed things down. Some colleagues saw HAZ work as an additional burden, rather than as integral to local activity. All HAZs were asked, as part of their plans, to request the freedoms they would like in order to achieve their aims. All HAZs submitted requests but there has been a lack of government response to some of these, which is disappointing. The general uncertainty over HAZ funding throughout their expected lives is making planning problematic. An adjournment debate in the House of Commons records that ministers were concerned that HAZs had underspent their budgets, but MPs in HAZ areas explained this was due to prudent planning to ensure initiatives were robust.

The policy context and government requirements of HAZs changed during the programme, as the government refined its priorities and new ministers brought their own perspectives. Since late 1999 there has been a strong emphasis on improving health and social care services, and integrating HAZs with mainstream NHS policy and action. The impact of this has still to be evaluated, but it is likely that in some areas the focus may have shifted away somewhat from concerted efforts to attack the root causes of ill health, in order to fund and accelerate the agenda of service modernization.

Along with Education Action Zones and Employment Zones, HAZs are examples of policy initiatives aimed, to greater or lesser extent, at geographical areas of deprivation. Such programmes are not new, in the sense that policy-makers have often adopted an area-based approach, particularly in the 1960s and 1970s (see Russell, this volume). There is much that the HAZ initiative might learn from the experience of past policies such as Education Priority Areas, the Urban Programme, community development projects, and so on (Allinsky, 1969; Higgins, 1978). For example:

- Citizen or community participation was often a key focus of these programmes but was used as a substitute for more radical action, was often tokenistic and was aimed at getting more from communities, over-estimating their ability to solve their own problems.
- There was often a focus on improving service delivery, to manage the poor more efficiently rather than act upon poverty.
- Resources for the programmes were marginal: for example, the Education Priority Areas took less than 1 per cent of the education budget; similarly, HAZ budgets are small compared with mainstream resources.
- Programmes had little impact either on national policy or on the material resources available to people.
- Such policies can suggest that social, economic or environmental problems are confined to the areas in question, and obscure the inequalities which are widespread in our society.

Although the HAZ programmes certainly need to support improvements in health and other local services, the best services in the world can only impact upon public health to a limited extent. To improve health, and especially to reduce inequalities, we will need to increase the effort directed at dealing with root causes of ill health, such as poverty, environmental and occupational hazards, poor housing, and social alienation.

CONCLUSION

There are many challenges facing HAZs. If their programmes are to help tackle inequalities, which is still a formal objective for HAZs and one to which many are deeply committed, they will need to act as effective agents for change. They must mobilize all possible local resources, as well as influencing national policy to support marginalized communities and provide decent incomes, living conditions and opportunities for all. What can be achieved at a local level will be limited unless there is a reorientation of national and, increasingly, international policies towards redistribution of wealth and power in favour of the poorest. Nonetheless, I believe that, at their best, many of the HAZs are demonstrating public health development work in action.

Some research into action zones has noted that staff with appropriate skills are very thinly stretched (LGA, 2000b), and that failures of institutional design at the top create stressful and unsustainable working conditions. It is important to have some continuity of staff in this kind of work, which is one of the most challenging areas of work in the public sector, so staff need to be nurtured and supported. The HAZ experience may provide lessons on the appropriate skills and knowledge needed in this area, which should also prove helpful in the development of multi-disciplinary public health teams.

HAZs must steer a careful path between government and local priorities, especially since the new emphasis on developing mainstream services may be at odds with local expectations. HAZs and other action zones must be allowed to make some mistakes if they are to be pioneers, and to share learning with others in a climate of trust and mutual co-operation.

Perhaps the greatest challenge will be to ensure that the successful elements of HAZ programmes are taken into the mainstream. This will require resource movement, cultural change and new partnerships. I do believe that the NHS should undertake public health and health promotion work, but unless there is defined and continued funding this will not happen except as marginal projects, while treatment and care services continue to take most resources. As the HAZs face both agendas, they will be at the sharp end of these debates.

Most HAZs believe, as we do, that their work is making an important difference to quality of life in their area. As part of our work, it is humbling to hear the very moving accounts of what the HAZ had achieved for people. It had provided motivation and resources for great need, which, in some cases, had been totally neglected before. Quite small amounts of cash and staff support have given people hope: hope that they could make a difference, that others cared about them, and that things could get better. My understanding and experience tell me that this is an essential element for improving health.

ACKNOWLEDGEMENTS

I am grateful to Keith Henshall and Colin Pollock for their help and advice.

5.2

OPPORTUNITIES FOR IMPROVING HEALTH THROUGH REGENERATION

Debs Harkins and Melissa Stead

Improving health has increasingly become an explicit objective of regeneration, as Hilary Russell has outlined above. Overwhelming evidence shows that those who experience material and social disadvantage have poorer health (Townsend and Davidson, 1982). Despite this, many still demand proof that regeneration initiatives benefit health, which assumes a simple 'cause and effect' relationship between deprivation and health. Anyone who has lived or worked in deprived communities knows that the relationship between health and poverty is complex. In this case study we outline some research undertaken in Sheffield to explore the relationships between health status and social and economic factors in two inner city areas undergoing integrated regeneration programmes.

The two areas received regeneration funding in 1995. One area obtained funding from URBAN and the other from the first round of the Single Regeneration Budget (SRB). Both included communities experiencing multiple deprivation, so that securing resources to undertake large-scale integrated regeneration was seen as a real opportunity to improve life for local people.

In February 1997 a team from the two universities in Sheffield was commissioned to carry out research which would establish a picture of what life was like in the two areas, to provide a baseline against which long-term change could be assessed. Part of the research involved a community survey, using face-to-face interviews with local people in their own homes, and undertaken by a team of interviewers recruited locally and trained in research skills. In the context of a regeneration programme, we felt it was important that the research resources contributed to the skills of local people and the local economy. The interviewers collected information on a range of social and economic issues, including health, and a full report is available giving a picture of these aspects of life in the two areas (Green et al., 1998).

Health status was measured using the SF-36, a series of survey questions which can reliably measure health within communities across a range of dimensions of health: physical functioning, role physical, role emotional, social functioning, pain, energy/vitality, mental health, self-perceived health and general health perception (Brazier et al., 1992; Jenkinson et al., 1996). The local health authority was keen to undertake a detailed analysis of the link between health status and other social and economic indicators to help understand the potential health opportunities offered by regeneration. To do this, we undertook a statistical analysis of the associations between SF-36 scores and other factors identified through the survey, such as housing, mobility, unemployment, fear of crime, social support and social exclusion. Below, we outline the relationships we observed between health and these other factors, and suggest how regenerating deprived communities could have a positive impact on health.

HOUSING

In both areas, we found that council tenants had significantly poorer health status than owner-occupiers. Tenure was related to physical health, mental health and self-perceived health. Unfortunately, it was not possible to show whether these were related to the quality of council housing. However, overall feelings about the home were related to mental health; the more dissatisfied with the home, the poorer the health state. It may well be that in these areas, people with poorer health were more likely to have been housed by the local authority, as the council prioritized housing people with a range of special needs including health needs. In both areas, the majority of the council housing was high rise flats and maisonettes, which have been shown to harm health in certain groups (Littlewood and Tinker, 1981; Lowry, 1990). Since we undertook the research the regeneration process has included significant improvements to the council housing in both areas, and building new properties managed through social landlords. The aim was both to reduce density and improve the quality of the accommodation, although reducing density has implications for household mobility and the social make-up of the community, as people are re-housed out of the area.

HOUSEHOLD MOBILITY

Area-based regeneration programmes are sometimes criticized on the grounds that those individuals who benefit from the initiatives are most likely to eventually leave the area. In terms of mobility, we found there were two distinct groups in the communities we studied. The first was of older people who had lived in the areas for many years and did not anticipate ever leaving, and the second was of younger people who considered themselves to be in the area temporarily. There were clear age-related health differences between these groups, with the second having significantly higher health status scores, particularly in the physical health and self-perceived dimensions of the SF-36. Those with poor health were far less likely to want to leave their area than those in better health, with the implication that as healthier people leave the proportion of those with poor health will increase, with a potentially detrimental effect on the social fabric of the area. With reductions in housing density, it is possible that fewer younger people will move into the area to replace those who leave. There is a clear role here for a public housing allocation policy which ensures that regeneration programmes create sustainable and self-supporting communities.

UNEMPLOYMENT

There is much evidence that people who are unemployed experience poorer health than those who are in paid work (Hakim, 1982; Bartley, 1994; Bartley et al., 1999), and our findings reflected this. Employment was related to all health dimensions, with those in full-time employment recording better health scores than those registered unemployed. The reasons for this are complex. Being out of work can have both material and psychological impacts, and it may also be that those with poorer health are more likely to lose their jobs or find it harder to gain employment. The regeneration programmes in the areas we studied have included the development of local training and skills centres and support for the development of community enterprises. The research process itself created employment, albeit temporary, for local people, many of whom then moved into employment or further/higher education. Strategies to increase marketable skills within the community, create jobs accessible to those living in deprived areas and reduce discrimination in the labour market should eventually have a positive effect on health through reducing unemployment.

FEAR OF CRIME AND TRUST

People in these areas believed that crime levels were higher than was actually the case. Being afraid of crime while at home was related to all dimensions of health status and was more common among older people. Feeling unsafe when walking alone after dark was also related to many of the health dimensions, even when age was taken into account. Fear of crime is associated with reduced quality of life and poor health (Audit Commission, 1999) and it has been argued that both ill health and crime have the same social origins (Kawachi et al., 1999). Fear of crime acts as an important barrier to participation in activities known to enhance health, such as community, physical or social activities outside the home. Regeneration programmes have a key role to play in reducing fear of crime. There are examples in some parts of the UK of housing improvement programmes which have included fitting security devices. Outside the home, improvements to the local environment such as better lighting, trimmed hedges and even closed circuit TV have increased residents' feelings of security. Such initiatives are most effective where local people are involved in identifying problems and solutions. For example, the Mansfield Community Safety Project in Nottinghamshire worked with local people and relevant agencies on estate audits to identify crime and safety 'hotspots'. The solutions included both environmental and social interventions. A number of 'New Deal for Communities' initiatives in the UK include the introduction of neighbourhood wardens to encourage local confidence about safety (Armstrong, 2000).

People's views about whether others can be trusted are related to fear of crime. A majority (60 per cent) of those we interviewed felt that people could generally be trusted, and they tended to be in better health than those who felt otherwise. Perceptions about local people and the local community will inevitably be complex and related to a range of personal beliefs and community characteristics. Deprived communities often have a high turnover of residents so that people may not even know their neighbours, let alone feel able to trust them. Comprehensive regeneration initiatives increasingly aim to improve both external and internal perceptions of deprived communities. Yet, however successful the regeneration programme, it may take many years to change negative views held within and about a deprived community. In one area of Sheffield with a long history of crime and instability, a regeneration programme prompted a housing association to prioritize the creation of a settled community in the hope that community confidence would grow (Social Exclusion Unit, 2000a). In North Nottinghamshire, one initiative aimed to build local confidence through a neighbour's calling card scheme in a community with high mobility.

SOCIAL SUPPORT AND EXCLUSION

Good social support and networks are associated with health (Campbell et al., 1999; Cooper et al., 1999; Stansfeld, 1999). We found that people who did not feel that their family and friends would help them out in a time of crisis had poorer health than those with faith in the support of their family and friends. Although fewer people felt that neighbours would help them out in a crisis, this feeling was also associated with better health. There are many examples of community development and health projects that aim to build social support in deprived communities, and the Coronary Heart Disease National Service Framework requires every health authority area to have at least one community development project working in a deprived neighbourhood (Department of Health, 2000a). Such projects can be most effective when they are linked to comprehensive regeneration programmes. Active, motivated and self-supporting communities stand to gain the most from regeneration programmes and it is no coincidence that the first stage of many recent initiatives has been the development of community capacity.

Feeling part of a community depends on having contact with others. We found that those who had frequent contact with their friends had better health than those with less social contact. The number of hours spent outside the home was also related to health: those who spent more time out of the house generally had better health status, irrespective of age. Although people who are already ill tend to spend more time in their homes, the fact that this indicator was related to all dimensions of health status shows that 'illness' alone cannot explain the association. People's ability to contribute to the everyday life of their community and wider society is enabled by employment, social networks and support, feeling secure and safe as well as by good health. We could debate cause and effect endlessly when talking of health and social exclusion, but an important challenge for regeneration programmes is to ensure that those with pre-existing poor health are just as able to benefit from improvements as anyone else.

CONCLUSION

A complex combination of social and economic factors affects the health of areas in need of regeneration. These factors cannot be isolated from one another to prove their relationship with health. Only a handful of the things that may influence health in deprived communities were measured in our survey, and many of the others are complex and difficult to quantify for statistical analysis. The implication of the research is that initiatives to improve housing, develop sustainable communities, create jobs, reduce fear of crime, increase social support, and develop community capacity may begin to reverse the trends of worse health in poorer areas. Such initiatives fall within the remit of a range of agencies and the role of the health service is to encourage, and engage in, partnerships to invest in health enhancing regeneration activities and to establish the health impact of regeneration plans. Within the current paradigm of 'effectiveness', there is strong pressure to justify NHS investment in such partnerships, but it may be many years before we can prove that regeneration is health enhancing unless we use intermediate indicators of impact, such as numbers of people in fear of crime, unemployment, participation in community activities, contact with others, and so on (Lindholm and Rosén, 2000).

There are many examples of projects where regeneration activities should contribute to a community's health, but it is important to recognize that improved health is both a cause *and* a consequence of regeneration. Integrated regeneration programmes need to ensure that those in poor health are not excluded from their benefits.

5.3

HEALTH AND LOCAL FOOD INITIATIVES

James Petts

FOOD AND INEQUALITY

The transformations which have industrialized agriculture and turned food into just another commodity have destroyed local economies, poisoned lands and rivers, and handed control of food to multi-national corporations. Increasingly, the food system is directed towards packaged, processed and out of season food. Nutrition, animal welfare, cultural diversity and taste have been sacrificed for uniformity, standardization and profit. Food now travels from the most distant parts of the globe, at the same time burning up fossil fuels, creating pollution, increasing the need for packaging and preservation, and reducing freshness and nutritional content. Inequalities in access and affordability of food, which follow from wider social inequality, contribute to the differences in health and longevity between rich and poor.

According to the United Nations Development Programme, Britain is one of the most unequal industrialized countries in the world (UNDP, 1996), and one reason for the poor health suffered by those on the lowest incomes may be because they find it difficult to obtain a healthy balanced diet. The National Food Survey (MAFF, 1997) shows that the average fresh green vegetable intake of large, poor families is equivalent to fewer than ten Brussels sprouts per person per week, and their fresh fruit consumption is equivalent to fewer than two apples per person per week. The World Health Organisation recommends at least five portions of fruit and vegetables per person per day.

Food poverty manifests itself in many different ways. People without the disposable income to afford fresh food face real difficulties in maintaining an adequate nutritional intake and healthy diet (Dobson et al., 1994). Price differentials encourage those on low incomes to consume heavily processed foods, high in fat, salt and sugar, such as cakes and biscuits, which are proportionately cheaper per calorie than fresh, sustainably produced food. Poor quality food has become the *only* food stocked in some local shops or 'budget' supermarkets, turning many deprived areas into 'healthy food deserts' – areas where affordable healthy food is difficult to find. In areas where a retailer has a local monopoly food prices will often be higher – further penalizing low income and disadvantaged groups. Low income households living in affluent areas are also vulnerable because food prices can be higher, so an increased proportion of the household budget is spent on food. In addition, people in all income groups may face practical problems in getting access to healthy food, especially if they are disabled, elderly, lack a car or live in an isolated rural community. Local food initiatives can offer only limited solutions to the problems, and local, regional and national strategies that seek to improve food security and increase access to good food are prerequisites to reducing food poverty.

REGENERATION AND LOCAL FOOD INITIATIVES

There are very many local food initiatives around the UK, and they take a wide variety of forms. Although they account for only a small fraction of the total food economy, the total turnover of farm shops, pick your own schemes, allotments and community gardens, food co-ops, farmers' markets and box schemes, breakfast clubs, community cafés, school nutrition groups, and so on, is probably substantial. Such initiatives may have simply commercial motivations or develop from community activities such as environmental, health or educational initiatives, or from money advice centres, credit unions or local exchange trading schemes. Different schemes carry different advantages and disadvantages, and their effectiveness in health terms has rarely been formally evaluated.

Although many Single Regeneration Budget and New Deal for Communities programmes have promoted housing and employment schemes, few have been involved with food accessibility. Some health authority schemes have attempted to promote healthy eating, but have mainly focused on dietary education and have failed to consider the bigger picture. Some have treated the symptoms rather than the causes of food poverty and insecurity, focusing on the individual rather than taking a collective approach (Caraher, Chapter 2.1, this volume). Others have taken a more holistic approach, starting or supporting local projects and regional networks, and have been successful in improving food security and sustainability. The voluntary sector and local communities themselves have usually been unsuccessful in gaining funds directly from regeneration budgets, due in part to a lack of awareness and resources.

The Plymouth Healthy Cities project recognized the connection between poverty and poor nutrition and set up a network to co-ordinate the local food initiatives in the area. These included an allotment group keen on organic gardening, two food co-ops, a couple of community cafés in deprived areas and the school meals service, among others. An initiative in East London helped the mainly Bengali residents to set up a food co-op in an area with poor access to fresh, affordable food, jointly funded by the health authority, local authority environmental health department, and Single Regeneration Budget money. Although the food co-op was not entirely successful, it did lead the participants to set up a food-growing project and then a cooking club and community catering enterprise. Some of the different types of local food initiatives are discussed below.

Growing initiatives

Community food-growing projects are attempting to address problems of food access and health inequalities. For example, Beacontree Organic Growers in

Dagenham aims to produce fresh, organic food locally at a price affordable to people on low incomes. Some projects link their activities to local food co-ops. Residents in Tipton were assisted by local conservationists to plant herbs and fruit trees in their gardens, taking what they wanted and selling the rest to the Sandwell food co-op at wholesale prices.

Although there have been very few studies of the health and nutritional benefits of 'growing your own', there is much anecdotal evidence to suggest that those who do have better access to fresh food, improved diets, and better mental and physical health. The mainly Bangladeshi community involved in the 'Gardening for Health' project in Bradford increased their intake of fresh vegetables as a result (Garnett, 1996). They also gained improved fitness, increased confidence and reduced food spending, because their traditional foods, which had to be imported, were very expensive. In one survey allotment holders felt that gardening and growing food helped their health, diet and fitness (Saunders, 1993). Two-thirds of respondents cited exercise and increased consumption of fresh vegetables as their main gains from allotment gardening.

One US study, of the Philadelphia Urban Gardening Project, found that gardeners ate significantly more dark green leafy vegetables and generally more of other vegetables too, and consumed less dairy produce, confectionery and sweet drinks (Blair et al., 1991). Another project in the USA sought to produce all the nutritional needs of one person from a 4,500 square foot plot. The garden yielded an average of 2,900 calories a day and all the nutrients required with the exception of vitamin B_{12}, and green leafy vegetables and potatoes provided the maximum nutritional benefit for the least labour (Knight, 1997).

Box schemes and farmers' markets

There is growing awareness of the damage caused by the existing food economy and a desire to develop 'local food for local people'. Box schemes can be run by farmers themselves, commercial distributors, or food co-ops, who supply food direct to the door, usually on a weekly basis. Some also try to source all their food locally. Farmers' markets enable consumers to buy direct from producers. Although many operate in the open market, tending to cater for middle and high-income groups, some have recognized the difficulty for people on low incomes. Green Ventures in South London has a 'sliding scale' of prices, calculated according to people's income, for its boxes of fresh fruit, vegetables, eggs and bread. Wheatlands farmers' market, inspired by a US Department of Agriculture scheme, plans to issue food vouchers to nutritionally 'at risk' groups in East London. The vouchers can be used at local farmers' markets, and farmers can redeem the vouchers for cash so that producers and consumers both gain.

Community cafés and shops

Community cafés offer a place where people can eat a nutritious, inexpensive meal in a social setting. They often develop as a meeting place for local people, especially vulnerable groups, and can act as a point of access for health professionals or provide information about education and employment opportunities.

Community shops are not-for-profit shops, such as a grocery, serving low income, isolated or 'housebound' shoppers. They can also act as an important social focal point, especially in isolated districts. Many encourage healthy eating by promoting weekly menus that favour healthy foods on a budget.

Breakfast and lunch clubs

Breakfast clubs usually offer a breakfast service to school children. Children who eat breakfast tend to be more active and have fewer weight problems, and teachers report that children tend to concentrate better on their work and truancy is reduced when breakfast is also offered to parents. Lunch clubs provide lunches to older adults and disadvantaged groups. They are usually run by the local authority, Women's Royal Voluntary Service, or a local Age Concern group. As well as good food, participants benefit from the social contact and support that go with lunch.

Food co-ops

Setting up a food co-op allows people to buy food in bulk, direct from wholesalers or farmers. By pooling their purchasing power, co-op members can save money on their food bills and can access healthier, better quality foods. In some areas, the food is delivered by the co-op to disabled, older or housebound members. Food co-op members gain substantial financial savings – often amounting to a third to a half of local shop prices – as well as increased consumption of fruit and vegetables.

Food co-ops are usually run by volunteers, which often means that they rely heavily on a small group of committed people. This may cause problems of continuity, limit the involvement of people with full-time jobs, and 'burn out' key members. The Sandwell food co-op in the West Midlands has avoided such problems, mainly through the size and structure of the group. As a network of 31 different outlets, it is able to supply cheap, fresh fruit and vegetables to hundreds of local residents who could not otherwise afford or have access to them. It has also started to grow its own food on allotment sites and community gardens, as well as buying food grown by local people in their own gardens.

PROBLEMS AND OPPORTUNITIES IN POLICIES AND REGULATIONS

International policies have an important impact on food and society. Decisions taken at meetings of the World Trade Organisation or the World Bank may seem a long way from most people's everyday life, but they affect domestic prices, incomes and policies, and shape the profile of the food economy. Market liberalization, structural adjustment policies, the growth of transnational corporations, and misguided development projects such as the 'green revolution' have often been to the detriment of people's health and diets, and particularly harmful to disadvantaged and vulnerable groups. Reform of these policies and institutions is necessary to improve food access and security.

Changes in the Common Agricultural Policy and other EU policies are also required. Agricultural subsidies related to production volumes have benefited large producers, which have swallowed up many small family farms (SAFE Alliance, 1998). More assistance for small-scale horticultural enterprises in urban areas and isolated rural communities could dramatically increase the availability of fresh, local produce.

National, regional and local government legislation and planning guidance could clearly do more to overcome health and food inequalities. By limiting large 'out of town' supermarket developments, encouraging food retailing in deprived neighbourhoods and protecting allotment sites and greenbelts, governments could help redress some of the problems with the food system and help develop local economies.

While local food initiatives can help solve some of the problems caused by the globalization of the food economy, they can only ever account for a small part of the total food system. They are not a panacea for all the ills of society, but they can and do help people overcome some of the difficulties they face – and such initiatives will probably be an essential element of any future sustainable food system that respects the environment and seeks to reduce inequalities in health and nutrition.

6

PUBLIC SERVICES AND HEALTH

Dexter Whitfield and James Munro

In the UK, the health promotion profession finds itself working within the structures of the National Health Service, an institution which in turn has as one of its purposes 'to secure improvement in the physical and mental health of the people of England and Wales' (Great Britain Parliament (1946) National Health Service Act, 1946). This historical optimism, which seems never to have quite been abandoned by politicians, even today, makes it easy to forget that the role of public services in protecting and improving public health goes far beyond both health promotion specialists and health services. In this chapter we briefly make the case, which, in the current climate of globalization and corporatization, can no longer be taken for granted, for the importance of public services to public health promotion, before going on to examine some of the threats to vigorous, effective and equitable public services. We conclude by discussing some of the necessary conditions for truly health enhancing public services.

That the health of each of us is critically dependent upon the health of others has long been understood as both a moral truth – 'no man is an island, entire of itself' (Donne, 1624) – and also, since at least the cholera epidemics of the nineteenth century, as a practical one (Chadwick, 1842). In recent times the emergence of new communicable diseases, such as HIV and BSE, and the reappearance of old ones, such as tuberculosis, coupled with increasing awareness of the health impacts of environmental quality (see Secrett and Bullock, Chapter 2, this volume) and of social inequality and injustice (see Duggan, Chapter 4, this volume) have continued to confirm the impossibility of securing health for some without securing health for all.

The role of the state in regulating economic activity and providing services in order to protect and promote the health of citizens (and particularly of the labour force required by industry and commerce) developed throughout the second half of the nineteenth and first half of the twentieth centuries in all industrialized nations, as it became widely understood that this was something which capitalist enterprise alone was unable or unwilling to do.

All industrialized nations now guarantee entitlement to at least some level of education, health care, housing and income support as of right, although of course the amount of provision, and the organization and funding of such services, differ widely between countries. Such provision is important to health in at least three different ways.

First, and most obviously, the direct effect of a public service may in itself be health enhancing, whether it is the result of explicit health promotion activity, or of other services which support and promote health, such as education (Beattie, Chapter 6.1, this volume), public transport (Public Health Alliance, 1991), housing (Lowry, 1991), income support (Abbott and Hobby, 1999), and so on. There is much evidence to suggest that improvements in living conditions, rather than in health services, have accounted for most of the gains in population health over the past two centuries (McKeown, 1979), although there is also evidence that preventive and curative medical care have contributed substantially to life expectancy during the twentieth century (Bunker et al., 1994). Either way, public services have made an important contribution to improving both material living conditions and health care.

Second, the equitable and universal provision of public services constitutes a guaranteed entitlement which stands, in Nye Bevan's famous phrase, 'in place of fear' (Bevan, 1952). Our health and sense of well-being benefit simply by knowing that services will be available – and that they will be available not only for ourselves, but for our family, friends and neighbours – without having to worry about whether we will be able to pay at the time we need them.

Third, the existence of public services is an important expression of social solidarity, of the responsibility that a society takes collectively for all of its members, irrespective of status or wealth. Public services aim to, and often do, respond to their users on the basis of need, not wealth, income or status. At best, therefore, public services embody the ideal that each of us is to be valued, not as a consumer or a producer in a marketplace, but simply as a human being. They offer an alternative to the values of the market – and this may be one reason why governments of the right are so often hostile to them.

Unfortunately, it is often true that public services fail to live up to the ideals we have for them. Education may be provided inequitably, social care inaccessibly, income support inflexibly and health care insensitively. Public services are far from perfect, yet at least there is the possibility of accountability and improvement, and of moving in a direction which takes us closer to the equitable, accessible, flexible and responsive ideal.

But what do we mean by 'public' services? In recent years, politicians in many countries have argued that it is enough for public services to be *paid for* by government, while the service providers can, or should, be in private *ownership*. Britain's Prime Minister, Tony Blair, has famously argued that 'what matters is what works', indicating an 'ideology-free' stance towards the continuing public ownership of services, which is seen as irrelevant. Is it really necessary for public services to be owned as well as paid for by government, if private services can simply be regulated for public ends? We would argue that it is, for economic, social and political reasons.

First, there is a clear economic argument in favour of public ownership. A range of evidence suggests that commercial services may frequently cost more, yet offer less (for example, Duckett, 2001; Shaoul, 1996). This should not be surprising, since of course for-profit providers must provide both a given level of service and, in addition, dividends for their shareholders.

Second, there is a political problem in controlling private providers and holding them to account. Privatizing the ownership of public services risks losing any effective democratic control over how, and what, services are

provided. Commercial service providers inevitably have interests and obligations – for example, to pursue profit-maximizing strategies – which will often or
always conflict with those of users and the community. Carefully designed regulatory regimes and funding systems can go some way towards controlling
behaviour of commercial providers in line with public policy goals. However,
the incentives and values of a private provider will always be different from
those of a public sector provider of services, and even the cleverest schemes for
financing such providers can never entirely escape the possibility of creating
perverse incentives, which promote behaviour which may be the opposite of
that intended (Harrison, 1991). The difficulties of achieving public policy objectives through complex contractual arrangements have long been demonstrated
by the 'independent contractor' status of primary care doctors in the NHS (Iliffe
and Munro, 1993) and more recently by the UK's ill-fated attempt to create an
internal market within a public health care system (Munro and Iliffe, 1997). For
public services to achieve their real potential as a force for individual and population health, 'high trust relationships' between communities and their
services – and among service providers themselves – are essential. Such relationships are constantly undermined in a competitive environment (Harrison
and Lachmann, 1996).

Third, there is a social cost to the privatization of public services. As we
have noted above, and as Campbell argues (Chapter 6.2, this volume), the relationship of each of us to the public services – particularly the caring services – is
one based on the twin ideas of trust and entitlement. Because the services are
provided without profit motive, we trust that they act, broadly, in our interests
when we need them, and we also recognize our entitlement, as citizens, to make
use of them when we need to do so. Such a relationship is immediately placed
at risk when the service is privatized, since we recognise new financial motivations on the part of the provider – a point which was central to the widespread
public concern over the GP fundholding policy. In addition, our position of entitlement as a citizen becomes subtly altered, so that we become simply another
paying customer, albeit paid for by the state. While we retain an entitlement, we
have lost our stake in the service, which is no longer a tangible expression of
social solidarity.

THE 'MARKETIZATION' AGENDA 1979–97

The strategy of the 1979–97 Conservative governments towards public services
was underpinned by a number of objectives including the transfer of ownership
of some services to the private sector; marketization of remaining public services; transformation of labour processes and reduction in the power of trade
unions; lower public expenditure in order to allow personal and corporate taxation to be reduced; maximization of opportunities for profit by deregulation;
creation of a smaller, more efficient and better managed state; and centralizing
power, under the guise of rolling back the frontiers of the state (Whitfield, 2001).

During this period the National Health Service bore the brunt of many of
these changes. For example, user charges rose repeatedly: NHS prescription
charges rose from 20p in 1979 to £6.10 by 2001, dental charges increased steeply

with non-exempt patients paying 80 per cent of the cost of NHS dental check-ups and treatment, and funding for sight tests was withdrawn in 1989. Paradoxically, despite remaining in public ownership the NHS became the single largest supplier of private health care in Britain, with revenue from private patients increasing by 230 per cent between 1979/80 and 1995/96. In 1991 the government undertook a radical experiment in marketization with the introduction of an 'internal market' in the NHS, in which service providers were constituted as separate 'trusts' which contracted with publicly funded purchasing authorities to provide care for defined populations. While the object was to improve efficiency and responsiveness, and possibly to prepare the ground for a full-scale privatization of the NHS in the future, many critics argued that the increasing bureaucracy and regulation which resulted had the opposite effect (Munro and Iliffe, 1997).

MODERNIZATION UNDER LABOUR'S 'THIRD WAY'

The election of a Labour Government in 1997 brought fundamental change, at least to political rhetoric. The new government constantly emphasized the importance of public services: 'the big fundamentals that determine our future – the economy, jobs, public services . . . we are doing the right thing' (Blair, 2000). Although New Labour's 'third way' was claimed to be distinct from the traditional policies of both the old left and the new right, in reality it turned out to look more like a patchwork of policies with no clear or coherent underlying philosophy, and showed strong continuities with the policies of the preceding Conservative administration (Harrison, 2001; Powell, 1999).

The Prime Minister claimed that 'our education, health and transport plans represent the most radical reform in public services over ten years any Government has produced since the war', but his vision of 'public services' was dishonest, or at least misleading. Despite its stated commitment to 'an NHS free at the point of use', Labour continued to support the gradual erosion of public ownership of the services and facilities on which the NHS depended, through the Private Finance Initiative and the 'concordat' with the private sector announced in late 2000 (Department of Health, 2000b). As we have argued above, the public ownership of public services is an important part of ensuring the efficiency, accountability and equity of service provision.

Although public sector capital investment was belatedly increased, Britain's infrastructure became increasingly owned and operated by multinational companies and financial institutions as a result of Labour's continued support for the Private Finance Initiative. The result was the progressive privatization of the health and social care infrastructure as new hospitals, information technology, residential homes, GP surgeries and medical centres and primary health facilities were financed by private rather public investment (see, for example, Pollock et al., 1999; Pollock et al., 2001). By mid-2001, 180 PFI schemes had either been signed or were at various stages of planning or procurement in the NHS in England, with a capital value of £7.4bn and a total cost of £10.6bn. In addition, the Department of Health was committed to investing £175m over the following four years in the NHS Local Improvement Finance

Trust (LIFT), a joint venture with Partnerships UK plc to own and lease health centres, surgeries and other parts of the 'primary care estate'. Both Conservative and Labour governments have claimed that a clear distinction can be drawn between the core medical activities and privately provided facilities management and support services in order to retain direct public employment of doctors and nurses, although in practice there is much evidence to contradict this (Whitfield, 2001).

Labour's claim that 'what works is what matters' indicates a lack of principled opposition to the increasing involvement of the private sector in public services, with the result that business interests are progressively replacing the public interest. Worthwhile innovations in services are being compromised by the preoccupation with involving business interests in everything from service design, delivery and development to regeneration and core welfare state functions. The 'three Ps' of partnership, procurement and private investment have become the mantra, as social and community needs have been downgraded or dropped entirely (for example, Walker, 2000).

Despite claims to be renewing democracy, there has been no fundamental attempt to improve the democratic accountability of the NHS and indeed the opposite may be the case, as Campbell argues in this volume. Health service organizations are effectively run as quangos, community health councils are to be abolished or radically reformed and the cabinet system in local government (centralized control in the hands of a few behind closed doors) does not bode well for joint health and social services initiatives. Although there have been some important initiatives in patient and NHS frontline staff involvement, focus groups, polls and panels have become the norm to elicit the views of users. However, such mechanisms do not give service users or local communities any formal power in the system.

Market testing or 'compulsory competitive tendering' has rightly been abolished but has been replaced by an even stronger commitment to procurement and market-driven services under a regime known as 'Best Value'. Wage cuts imposed on mainly women workers through contracting out may achieve a marginal reduction in support service budgets but risk increasing health inequalities and impose other costs on the NHS and the public sector. Local authorities must now 'develop markets' where there is little or no history of outsourcing, for example, in social services. Many NHS estates departments and computer services have been sold off to the private sector.

These changes to Britain's welfare services are part of a larger global movement towards opening up public services to corporate investment. The World Trade Organisation's negotiations on General Agreement on Trade in Services (GATS) represent a fundamental threat the NHS (Pollock and Price, 2000; Sexton, 2001). The objective of the WTO and the multinational business interests promoting it, including health and drug companies, is to create a worldwide market in all public and private services. GATS will facilitate trade in services across national borders by requiring WTO member countries to treat all countries the same – treating foreign companies as if they were domestic ones. This will impose severe restrictions on the ability of governments to maintain public ownership of public services or to protect public health. GATS represents an enormous deregulation initiative to marketize and privatize

public services in every country, without exception. The current round of negotiations is planned for completion by December 2002.

When Tony Blair promised 'a second term more radical than the first' in his
Brighton conference 2000 speech, he was sending a message to the private sector
that the next five years will see a fundamental shift towards marketization and
privatization under the banner of 'public services'. Public funding and provision
have led to the NHS being one of the most efficient health care systems in the
world. The NHS spends less than 12 per cent of its budget on administrative
costs – up from 6 per cent before the Tories introduced the internal market. This
is in stark contrast to the 23-34 per cent administrative costs of public and private hospitals in the USA where 44m people cannot afford health insurance
(Himmelstein and Woolhandler, 1986). In Australia, public hospital administrative costs are 31 per cent less than those for private hospitals. The implication is
that plans to raise health expenditure may not improve the services users
receive, because marketization and privatization will increase the share of the
budget spent on administration and overhead costs.

The government's social inclusion strategy and reform of the welfare state
are attempting to reduce inequalities. Health action zones, welfare to work and
the New Deal for Communities are important elements of this strategy, but
questions remain over whether they can achieve their objectives or whether
they will further fragment service delivery. A major question concerns the
longer-term effects of increasingly transferring risk and responsibility for welfare
and pensions from the public to the private sector and individuals, personaliz-
ing social needs and the commodification of risk. The restructuring of the NHS
and local government has had a major impact on patients, staff and services.
Rather than reduce or eliminate inequalities, the marketization and privatization
'reforms' of public services undermine the ability of services to be truly health
promoting, and make the achievement of public health goals more difficult.

AN ALTERNATIVE MODERNIZATION STRATEGY

Despite the narrow modernization agenda, creeping privatization through
charges, concordats and private finance, business-oriented policy-making and
uncritical acceptance of the WTO agenda shown by current politicians, there are
still opportunities for radical change, particularly in the interface between health
and other related services.

An alternative modernization agenda is urgently needed, with a focus on
democratization, public health impact, public investment and management.
First, new local democratic structures and methods of accountability are
required for trusts and other health quangos, combined with the strengthening
of community health councils. The trend towards quangos and the regionaliza-
tion of health and social care in new unaccountable trusts should be reversed.
'Best Value' potentially offers new opportunities for patient and public involvement in health care planning and service performance plus cross-cutting reviews
such as services for the elderly, children and other groups. However, this
requires new ways to involve community and patient organizations and
employees, particularly frontline staff, and trade unions in the review process.

Professional barriers and protectionism must be broken down and services reconfigured to meet health and social care needs.

Democratization should be accompanied by resources for capacity building for community and civil society organizations concerned with health matters. Genuine participation requires financial support for training, consultation and technical expertise.

Second, genuine joined-up government is needed to ensure health care is planned, managed and delivered as an integral part of regeneration and social inclusion, joint commissioning of health and social care, housing, education and lifelong learning. Joined-up government must avoid 'take-over competitions' between the NHS and local government about who is ultimately responsible for health and social services. There is also considerable scope for a wider range of community health projects to test new approaches to health promotion and primary care.

At the same time, health impact analysis should be integrated into social and economic auditing of public sector budgets and policies. All public policies should be assessed for their health implications as part of the planning process. The principles of equality and social justice should become central to health promotion, health and social care planning, management and service delivery. This should embrace equalities for services users and those employed in health and social care organizations. Equity audits should be accepted as an integral part of assessing the performance of all services, functions and organizations.

Third, increased public investment is urgently required in the health and education infrastructure, alongside with the abolition of the Private Finance Initiative. This is affordable. Although the government has increased public spending both overall and specifically for health, the public finances remain financially strong. The government had a £16.4bn surplus in 2000/2001 (Inland Revenue tax revenue was £6bn higher than expected and social security costs were £2bn lower than forecast) and further surpluses were forecast in subsequent years. The debt-to-GDP ratio fell to 32 per cent in 2000/01, well below the Treasury's prudent target of 40 per cent and the Maastricht convergence criteria of 60 per cent. Furthermore, Labour's commitment to increase health expenditure to the OECD average ignored the years of under-investment and current social need, particularly in inner city and rural areas. Recent policy announcements suggest that the government may now be prepared to consider raising taxes specifically to increase public funding for health care.

Fourth, a commitment to direct provision is essential to increase the capacity of health organizations. There is mounting evidence that it does matter who delivers the service. Achieving health targets and outcomes is important but the processes by which health services are delivered are inherent to the quality of care. An increasing proportion of health resources are tied up in inter-organizational coordination, contracting and administration rather than service delivery. Partnerships in health must focus on achieving added value rather than merely replacing in-house provision with private firms and voluntary organizations.

Accordingly, a new public service management must replace the competition and commercial-dominated performance management. It should focus on the effectiveness of services, investment and the process of provision, not just on results; participatory governance, not mere consultation; commitment to the improvement of in-house services by redesign and valuing staff, not by out-sourcing or making markets; accountability to users, civil society and staff, not merely to business; and integrated management and organizational structures, not divisive separation of purchaser and provider functions. Rebuilding state capacity is essential to provide a viable alternative to private sector management and dependency on management consultants. Alongside this, the re-regulation of the private and voluntary health and social care sectors is necessary to prevent the emergence of a two-tier care system, although the regulatory regime should not inhibit innovation and the development of new approaches. Finally, on the global stage our government, with others, should increase its opposition to GATS by re-emphasizing the importance to health of public services which are effective, efficient, accountable and truly accessible to those who need them most.

6.1

EDUCATION FOR SYSTEMS CHANGE:
A KEY RESOURCE FOR RADICAL ACTION
ON HEALTH

Alan Beattie

EDUCATION AND HEALTH, BEYOND THE FRAGMENTS

World-wide, schools have long been a vital resource in broader national strate-gies for protecting and improving public health, and some conspicuous advances in health have been made through work in education settings. A first priority is usually to ensure adequate physical environments for learning, and from the late 1800s public health advice played a prominent part in school build-ing policies and programmes (Beattie, 1996). Schools have also long been an important venue for taking action on some of the worst features of deprivation in pupils' backgrounds, for example, by providing school milk, school meals (breakfasts, dinners) and after-school facilities (homework clubs); and child health services are another element of social welfare provision that makes use of school settings (Armstrong, 1993). From the 1970s onwards in the developed world, schools became test-beds for exploring ways of delivering health educa-tion focused on lifestyle issues. Drawing on socio-psychological insights into child and adolescent development, systematic and coherent programmes were devised for different ages and stages, typically employing active, interactive and experiential pedagogies to guide pupils' personal and social learning (Weare, 1992).

But by the early 1990s (both in the UK and elsewhere) such child-centred personal-social-health education in schools was coming to look less stable – sometimes taken-for-granted and marginalized, and increasingly beleaguered (Chitty and Simon, 1994). It was shouldered aside largely by 'core curriculum' policies, embedding new ideologies of vocational preparation and credentialing for the 'information society', and by greater readiness to individualize blame and to regard troubled pupils as 'culpable unfortunates'; and soon the numbers of pupils excluded from schools – whether officially, or informally (by truancy, disaffection, or disengagement) – began an inexorable rise (Parsons, 1999).

At the beginning of the new millennium, public policy on 'education and health' remains fragmented and confused. Both the continuing contribution of schools to public health, and also the health impact of the growing emphasis on learning beyond the school, are crucial test-cases for intersectoral policy. An urgent and fundamental rethink is needed of the vital contribution that education can make to achieving greater equity and social inclusiveness in health. There are no easy and instant solutions, but at least three domains of research and development offer promise of more 'joined-up' policies and practice. These 'leading edge' areas all focus on education as a catalyst for systems transformation.

SCHOOLS AS SUPPORTIVE ENVIRONMENTS FOR HEALTH

The 'health promoting school' (HPS) has been one of the key exemplars of the WHO's linked concepts of 'healthy settings' and 'supportive environments for health' (World Health Organisation, 1993). This policy has helped to legitimate and encourage a unified approach, combining:

- teaching and learning about health matters that happens in classrooms;
- pastoral care and welfare support that the school can mobilize for individual pupils in need;
- nursing treatment and preventive medicine that pupils receive through school health services;
- the school as an institution: as a physical space and building, and as a community resource.

HPS projects can link environmental improvement and provision of child health services to cultural approaches that focus on pupil lifestyles and risk-taking behaviours, and they can also follow up what pupils learn in the classroom into and throughout the daily life of the school and well beyond, into the home lives of pupils. Numerous guidelines and standards for HPS have been developed – international, national, and local – and all of them emphasize the need to take action across all the different facets of school life (for example, Box 6.1.1).

Teachers need substantial support to implement HPS schemes, and public health/health promotion units can play a vital role in providing this. Investment in such work has been shown to yield significant gains: higher pupil self-esteem, healthier eating patterns, less bullying, less smoking and drinking, and also in some schools greater willingness to deal with staff health, particularly action on stress, and more involvement of parents and local community agencies. Perhaps most important of all is the growing realization that a health promoting school helps to foster exactly those features known to be characteristic more generally of 'the effective school' (Reynolds et al., 1993). It seems that when action for health unfolds across the whole school, it leads to shared school aims, higher expectations of pupils, and broad academic and social gains: 'healthy schools are effective schools' (Toft et al., 1996). A recent full-scale critical review commissioned by the UK government underlines the 'joined-up' action that successful HPS projects require:

> carefully and skilfully executed interventions following the HPS approach have the potential to improve children and young people's health. Given the relatively low cost of these interventions and their potential for improving health, further experimentation should be encouraged . . . The HPS initiative

BOX 6.1.1 AIMS OF THE EUROPEAN NETWORK OF
HEALTH PROMOTING SCHOOLS

Provide a health promoting environment for working and learning through
its buildings, play areas, catering facilities, safety measures, etc.
Promote individual, family and community responsibility for health.
Encourage healthy lifestyles and present a realistic and attractive range of
health choices for schoolchildren and staff.
Enable all pupils to fulfil their physical, psychological and social potential and
promote their self-esteem.
Set out clear aims for the promotion of health and safety for the whole school
community (children and adults).
Foster good pupil-pupil and staff-pupil relationships and good links between
the school, the home and the community.
Exploit the availability of community resources to support action for the promotion of health.
Plan a coherent health education curriculum with educational methods that
actively engage pupils.
Equip pupils with the knowledge and skills they need both to make sound
decisions about their personal health and to preserve and improve a safe and
healthy physical environment.
Take a wide view of school health services as an educational resource that can
help pupils become effective health care consumers.

Source: WHO, 1993.

> is new, complex and developing, and implementation of all the components
> may take several years in any one school. Studies of programmes combining
> the 3 domains of curriculum, school ethos and environment showed that
> these were more likely to be effective than those which did not. (Lister-Sharp
> et al., 1999: 24; 113)

Another major independent review (which focuses on literature from Australia
and the USA, and on primary schools specifically) comes to similar conclusions:
'health gains for primary school students . . . will most likely occur if a well-
designed program is implemented which links the curriculum with other
health-promoting school actions, contains substantial professional development
for teachers, and is underpinned by a theoretical model' (St Leger, 1999). St
Leger suggests that there is, by now, a high degree of commonality across different regions of the world in the structural frameworks being used to support
the 'multifaceted' approach to HPS work, amounting to a 'new theoretical paradigm', and that, if only one or two of the building blocks of the HPS approach
are employed, without understanding and applying more comprehensive
frameworks, the full benefits are not achieved.

A further review of all published evaluation studies (Beattie, 2001) –
including first-hand reports of HPSs in action, as well as these two secondary

critical reviews – highlights the importance of 'whole systems' thinking for a 'joined-up' approach to health action at school level (see Box 6.1.2).

BOX 6.1.2   LESSONS FROM THE EVALUATION OF HEALTH PROMOTING SCHOOL INITIATIVES

1   HPS projects must be about more than just health promotion 'based in' schools: they must be school-wide and strategic, focused on improving the school as a whole and as a resource for the community.

2   HPSs are most successful when activities are undertaken simultaneously, in parallel with one another, in several different domains (curriculum; environment; ethos; parent and community involvement): it may be helpful for local projects to put more emphasis on the 'capacity-building' that is entailed in connecting health promotion to other initiatives and other priorities in school improvement.

3   Not only is the curriculum element not enough on its own: in itself it must go beyond information-giving, and focus on health-related skills (e.g. assertiveness, coping, problem-solving), values, and cultural awareness.

4   Those developing and evaluating HPSs have not devoted as much attention to mental/emotional and social well-being as to physical health: local projects need to give greater priority to debating and negotiating these other goals of HPSs (including stress, morale, coping, school ethos), and strategies for achieving them.

5   HPSs have been quite successful in focusing on the health and lifestyles of pupils, but need to widen their horizons to give a higher profile to staff (their professional development and their health) and to the school as a workplace, both as a physical environment and as a social organization.

6   Planning and implementing HPSs have been most successful when there has been more involvement of pupils (peers), of parents and of external agencies in the local community: HPSs need to undertake such bottom-up partnership work to counter-balance the traditional top-down approach to planning and delivery.

7   Those involved with HPS projects need to acknowledge more fully the links between the healthy school and the effective school: to address explicitly how far and in what ways pupils' learning can be improved when effort is invested in improving health, and to clarify what counts as evidence of 'effectiveness' in the HPS.

8   Those involved with HPS projects need to make clear the theoretical basis of their interventions, and report fully and critically the approach or model(s) they are employing; and among all those with a stake in a HPS project (school staff, NHS staff, welfare staff, parents) there needs to be fuller and wider dialogue and debate to clarify what goals or

outcomes the HPS is seeking, and how these relate to the theoretical model(s) used.

9 There needs to be more appreciation of schools as complex systems, and a readiness to adopt and adapt more sophisticated theoretical models that can connect together both health concerns and criteria and educational concerns and criteria.

10 There needs to be more monitoring and evaluation of HPSs: it needs to be built into projects, and it needs to be more rigorous and creative, to take account of continuing debate about goals, processes and outcomes, and to illuminate these and other issues of theory.

The HPS is therefore a key project on which practitioners from health and education sectors can work together to deliver conjoint policies. In doing so, they can use a number of 'tools of thought' to get the multi-faceted approach firmly in place. Table 6.1.1 illustrates a specimen local interagency 'contract' for a HPS, showing the different strategies that need to be deployed simultaneously; each of them then unfolded across the several domains of corporate life in the school. A contract like this is above all a 'framework for dialogue': it can be used to prompt discussion of the different sorts of aims, purposes, procedures, targets (and underlying values and beliefs) that diverse stakeholders bring to any HPS project, and can help those involved to figure out which aims, activities and values they can agree on. It is a way of keeping the full menu of strategic choices in view.

ACTION LEARNING AND ORGANIZATION DEVELOPMENT IN HIGHER EDUCATION AND THE WORKPLACE

Recent policies have dramatically enhanced participation rates of young people in tertiary education, but have reduced the financial support they receive, making it imperative to ask how far colleges and universities act as 'supportive environments for health'. The health promoting college initiative in further education (O'Donnell and Gray, 1993) and health promoting campus projects in the university sector (Beattie, 1998) have begun to adopt some of the lessons learned from health promoting schools and other settings-based health promotion initiatives (Baric, 1993). Crucial to these lines of work is again the use of multi-faceted frameworks that seek wider 'systems change' through active, co-operative learning and campus-wide consultation and participation. This echoes broader shifts in favour of 'dialogical' and 'constructivist' approaches to learning in universities (Duffy and Cunningham, 1996). Such 'structured dialogue' has also become a familiar resource to many managers in workplace settings as a way of driving both individual staff development and systems change, to work towards 'empowered organizations'. Indeed the most fully-developed example of 'whole systems thinking' (Argyris and Schön, 1974) is probably the theory and practice that has evolved around 'the learning organization' (Senge, et al., 1999). This incorporates:

Table 6.1.1 A contract for multi-faceted, multi-level development in a health promoting school

Action	Curriculum content and pedagogy	Ethos staff/pupil relations; access to information and decisions	Environment physical space, facilities, support services	Institution structures and systems of decision-making and communications
Give information and advice – to redirect the behaviour of individuals and reduce personal risks to health	Talks, videos, seminars on current health topics and priorities	Clear information and guidance on how health risks and infractions of codes will be dealt with	Space and resources for health promotion; exhibitions, displays, events	Clear and decisive house rules and codes on risks e.g. smoking; safety; HIV/AIDS; alcohol; bullying; stress
Offer personal guidance and counselling – to support life-review and to strengthen individuals so as to encourage self-directed change	Individual support and pastoral care; discussion, role play, interactive work on peer pressures and social-and-life skills	Provision of opportunities and support for self-review and self-help; Informal ways of dealing with stress, 'corridor rage' and similar incidents in emotional life of school	Facilities for self-help and group work	Systems to support staff and pupils who need to adapt to rules and codes
Invest in outreach and liaison and networking – to identify common ground and strengthen community links and facilitate joint action	Courses for parents; links to adult and community education; Staff support; Challenge social exclusion in work with outside local agencies, and with voluntary self-help schemes	Set up local networks; increase community participation; improve communication: school–home and school–community; open meetings and events	Labelling, signposting, way-finding for all visitors; briefings on environmental awareness	Act as statutory enabler Create or maintain supportive networks and infra-structures: e.g. parent involvement; community service and volunteer schemes; visitor schemes
Take regulatory administrative action – to improve the environments: physical, social, cultural	Assignments and projects that link health issues to the school building and grounds, to the locality, and to global agendas on environment change	Give access to information and decisions about school environment and its impact on locality	Offer community use of school facilities; liaison over issues of school grounds, roads and car use, journeys to school; 'greening the school'	Lobby and campaign to transform local environments; laws, regulations, policies; standards, plans

- experiential learning, to help practitioners to engage directly in critical and creative reflection on their own work, to explore and challenge the mental models with which they work;
- team learning, to encourage interchange of experiences and building shared visions;
- action learning, and 'action learning sets', to help practitioners look for and implement changes in their current ways of working, in the light of individual and shared reflections.

Many in public health may be familiar (if only indirectly) with these lines of work as adopted in the whole systems approach to 'urban health partnerships' (Pratt et al., 1999), and as recommended in recent guidelines on Health Action Zones (Judge et al., 1999a, b). Such approaches emphasize that learning can be massively stimulated by starting from participants' work settings, with their own job-derived agendas of concern. Moreover, what can be learned from workplace experience encompasses much more than just technical knowledge or skills: if staff are to learn to embrace new options, new perspectives, new capabilities, and to learn to lead policy and practice in radically new directions, they must also expect personal change, and the development of new interpersonal relations within teams or across the organization. Learning of these kinds will often challenge the self-concept of the professional practitioner and must do so if it is to 'emancipate staff from tradition, precedent, habit, coercion or self-deception' (Kemmis, 1981). These approaches can again be seen as examples of 'dialogical' or 'dialectical' education: 'programmes that are put together in ways that boldly juxtapose different orientations to learning, so as to demand participants' attention to differing perspectives on what is educationally valuable may be particularly useful in encouraging professional flexibility and in preparing the "reflective practitioner"' (Beattie, 1990: 7; see Table 6.1.2).

Traditional practitioner	Reflective practitioner	Table 6.1.2 A comparison of two types of professional practitioner
I am presumed to know and must claim to do so	I am presumed to know much, as also is my client; my uncertainties may be a crucial source of learning	
I maintain a distance from my client	I work together with my client	
I expect deference and respect from my client	I prefer to have no mask of professional authority	
I expect the client to have faith in my expertise, and to put themselves in my hands	I expect to negotiate an interpretation and a plan through negotiation with my client	

Source: after Schön, 1983

Educational programmes constructed on dialogical/dialectical principles are better able to 'unfreeze' practitioners' taken-for-granted assumptions about definitions and justifications of learning – which are often the major source of resistance to organizational change (Figure 6.1.1). By encouraging debate about

Figure 6.1.1 A
fourfold dialectical
approach to
devising
professional
education

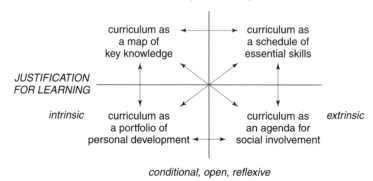

different starting assumptions and letting them interrogate and challenge each other, such programmes can enhance the flexibility and responsiveness of practitioners and of organizations and can help them to deliver radical agendas for change (Beattie, 1987).

PEDAGOGIES OF SOCIAL EMPOWERMENT IN ADULT AND COMMUNITY EDUCATION

Meanwhile, out on the streets, many volunteers and many professionals have worked hard since the late 1970s to enhance community involvement and get a hearing for the voices of lay people on health matters (Smithies and Webster, 1998), yet it is still not widely appreciated that community work and community development (in health and other areas of social welfare) have been hugely informed by the strategy of 'emancipatory education' or 'critical pedagogy' (Mayo, 1999). Derived from the literacy programmes of Freire (1972), such work entails setting up cycles of 'collective action-and-reflection' with social groups who are disadvantaged, disenfranchised, marginalized, or excluded, to help them to 'find a voice'. The Freire approach is essentially 'dialogical': learning is shared, active and experiential, and involves structured dialogue and mutual peer support. While much of this work has gone on in less developed countries (Craig and Mayo, 1994), it has also been extensively used in the UK, Australia, Canada and the USA, in 'radical adult education' (Brookfield, 1983) and 'health promotion through community development' (Wallerstein and Bernstein, 1988). Similar pedagogies of empowerment 'at the grassroots' can be seen (again, both in education and health settings) in 'participatory action research' (Nichter, 1984), such as 'participatory needs assessment' (Oladepo et al., 1991), and 'participatory evaluation' (Feuerstein, 1988).

Action-reflection learning cycles can bring professional staff (both from public health agencies and from local authorities) closer to local residents and community groups, and build up a powerful momentum for shared, locally owned work on all the different phases of action for health, as seen for example in the development of community education for mothers and children in deprived circumstances (Calder, 1984). It can be a uniquely successful way to articulate the health issues important to adults living on the margins, and to bring about personal and social transformation to tackle such issues (Jeffs and Smith, 1999). It is a vital element for a concerted approach to education-and-health in situations of oppression and deprivation (McLaren, 1995).

BORDER CROSSINGS: EDUCATION WITHOUT WALLS, HEALTH IN OPEN SPACE

Education and health are increasingly intertwined in multi-agency partnerships for urban regeneration. Schools are one crucial setting for the future development of sustainable public health, and their role will be greatly enhanced if they are seen as nodes in local lifelong-learning networks. Partner agencies need to be vigilant to ensure that academic and vocational pressures do not militate against this. They also need to invest in colleges, universities and workplaces as settings for health action through staff development and organizational learning. Outside the institutions, radical adult/community education is also a crucial vehicle for ensuring wide dialogue about 'whose needs count' and 'whose voices will be heard' in the struggle for health – to assist in processes of democratic renewal, and to counter the predatory culture of bureaucratic excess, media soundbites and tabloid headlines.

In the 1970s, person-centred health education was a source of countervailing arguments against biomedical dominance in public health policy and practice. Delivering the radical public health agenda now needs investment in the kinds of 'education for systems change' reviewed here. The many and diverse strands of this all emphasize constant switching between critical/reflective and creative/actionable ways of thinking, and between individual and collective agendas: not just learner-centred *but also* focused on transforming the social contexts in which health and life-chances are determined. Education along these lines is vital to challenge public health to jettison the mechanistic and cybernetic 'control and command' metaphors by which it is still too often dominated, and to replace them by metaphors more appropriate to the new global movements for social change: interconnection, interplay, multiple narratives, contested concepts, constructive conflict, complexity, fluidity, and self-renewal (Morgan, 1986; Urry, 2000). Public health needs to be allied with educational work that opens up spaces for conversation across ideological divides, and helps to construct the 'culture of dialogue' that may be the only way to resolve the contemporary dilemmas of governance and social policy – a vital feature of the politics of civil society (Cohen and Arato, 1992). Only through such alliances will public health play the part it should in the struggle to give practical reality to inclusive, participatory approaches to social policy, and 'deliberative' models of democracy and the public sphere (Calhoun, 1997).

6.2

PUBLIC SERVICES, PUBLIC HEALTH AND HEALTH PROMOTION: THE ROLE OF LOCAL AUTHORITIES

Fiona Campbell

The roots of the present health promotion movement in the UK are to be found in the work of the great nineteenth-century local government reformers on sanitation, waste disposal and public housing. At the time of their work, the links between poverty, the need for what we now call 'regeneration' and health were not in doubt. Over the twentieth century, recognition of those links was gradually eroded in public policy-making, so that for nearly two decades at the end of the century, we had a government that analysed the non-medical causes of ill health and health inequalities almost exclusively in terms of personal behaviour and individual choice.

With the election of a Labour government in 1997, the structural socio-economic causes of ill health were once again officially recognized. In his first speech as Secretary of State for Health, ranging widely over areas not notably associated by the previous government with ill health, Frank Dobson mentioned tobacco advertising, air pollution, food, homelessness, unemployment, low wages, poverty, crime and disorder. These are all areas in which local government has potentially an important role to play. Dobson pointed out that 'poor people, homeless people, jobless people and badly paid people are ill more often and die sooner. That is the greatest inequality of them all' (Hansard, 1997). In tackling poor housing, low wages and high unemployment and, thereby, poor health, he referred to the need for partnerships between central and local government, business and voluntary organizations.

Despite this early acknowledgement of the potentially central role of local government in health promotion and reducing inequalities, national government has shown a seriously ambivalent attitude towards local authorities. On the one hand, the government introduced, in the Local Government Act 2000, the power for local authorities to take action to address the 'social, economic and environmental well being' of the communities they serve, and a statutory duty on councillors to produce a 'community strategy' addressing the well-being of their communities. A strategy of this kind ought, by any common-sense analysis, to include strategic planning on issues that impact on health, since it is hard to imagine a community in a state of social, economic and environmental well-being that is not also in a state of good health.

Yet the government had already introduced, in the Health Act 1999, a on health authorities to work in partnership with local authorities in proc a health improvement programme for each locality. This duty was widel comed by both sides. Progressive public health and health promotion speciaŭ. welcomed it because it seemed to establish a forum in which local authorities could contribute more systematically to health improvement beyond their traditional social services role; and it created an opportunity to encourage a corporate approach to health across local authorities, breaking free of the traditional 'silos' of education, environment, housing and so on. Imaginative local authorities also welcomed the move as recognition of their contribution to health, and because they felt that they might now have greater influence in encouraging a health promotion approach in the NHS which was broader than the traditional disease-oriented model (Campbell, 2000). Less progressive (and cash-strapped) health and local authorities have been able to get away with allowing health promotion to take a back seat for many years. At their most positive, the well-being power and the duty of partnership taken together ought to provide an incentive for all health and local authorities to think seriously about resourcing work on health promotion and reducing health inequalities.

On the other hand, the government made it clear that health authorities were to take the lead in the development of the health improvement programmes and that they were to be dominated by national medically defined targets, for example, on coronary heart disease; this creates potential conflict with local authorities, which, with their direct links to local neighbourhoods and their overall strategic planning remit, remain the obvious facilitators of the new bottom-up community strategies.

In another initiative that alienated large numbers of elected local councillors, they were denied any statutory place on the newly-created primary care groups (PCGs) and trusts (PCTs), with a place in management structures offered only to one of their officers, in the case of social services authorities, and no place at all, in the case of district councils. None of these places is currently reserved for an elected councillor and there are no indications as to how lay members should be accountable to their supposed 'constituencies'. PCTs are, in reality, run on a day-to-day basis not by their boards but by their executive committees, with a majority of health professionals, one social services officer and no lay members other than the chair, an appointed nominee who is most unlikely to be an elected councillor.

Furthermore, the Health and Social Care Act 2001, through the introduction of care trusts, seriously weakens local democracy and accountability by removing direct responsibility for social care from local authorities. Councillors will be expected to delegate significant proportions of their budgets, as well as capital assets, to bodies over which they will have a minimal amount of influence. The Department of Health stated that 'local councils will remain ultimately accountable for the delegated services' (Department of Health, 2001). It is hard to understand how such accountability can be meaningful, given the governance arrangements proposed. In the case of local authorities, care trusts look like a serious case of responsibility without power.

Local authorities are also concerned that bringing social care under the NHS will inevitably (because of pressure on acute services) emphasize a narrow medical model of care for older and disabled people and people with mental health problems, which will undermine the holistic approach to social inclusion developed by local authorities and the voluntary sector, in response to the increasingly strong views of service users themselves. Concern about this issue was reinforced by Department of Health (2001) which states: 'The importance of the social model of care for people with learning disabilities ... may mean that this group may be best served by the local council taking the lead using Health Act flexibilities.' (That is, a care trust is not currently recommended for learning disabilities.) This statement strongly suggests both that the Department of Health does not understand the need for a social model of care for *all* client groups, and also that it does not believe that health bodies are equipped to operate such a model.

The statutory presence of social services officers on PCT executive committees, while worthwhile, seems to define the local authority contribution to health as simply professional social care, as does the creation of the significantly named 'care trusts'. This, of course, is completely at odds with a strategy of addressing the socio-economic causes of health inequalities. And, by failing to include elected councillors as equal partners as of right, it does nothing to reinforce the democratic role of local government.

WHY DOES DEMOCRACY MATTER IN HEALTH?

References to the 'democratic deficit' in health tend to be met with responses ranging from scorn to bewilderment by exponents of the new managerialism in public policy-making. In a recent discussion about the proposed power of scrutiny of health services by local government, a health authority chief executive said, 'If they set up a committee to scrutinize me, I'll set one up to scrutinize them.' This seems to me a clear failure to recognize the need for local accountability in health care. With their attitude that the only important thing is 'what works', it hardly seems to matter to such professional managers whether local communities or their elected representatives are involved in making decisions about health services and broader public health strategies.

As Will Hutton put it, in a report of a commission appointed by the Association of Community Health Councils for England and Wales, the NHS 'is perhaps the least accountable of Britain's major public institutions, even though access to health is the prime concern of British citizens' (Hutton, 2000: 8). Of all the 'quality of life' issues, health matters most to ordinary people. For this reason alone, they should have a say in decisions that will affect their health. But with health, in particular, 'having a say' should not just consist in voting for one party or another in a general election, on the basis of policies on NHS funding, waiting times for operations, and so on. Genuine consultation and participation in decisions about local health strategies can, in itself, make a difference to individuals' health, as work with poor communities in developing countries, and increasingly in the UK, has shown (Smithies and Webster, 1998; Hogg, 1999 and many studies in the journal *Health Expectations*).

Local authorities may not always have consulted and involved their communities in the most participatory and empowering way possible, but they certainly have a better track record than health authorities or, for that matter, general practitioners, who now have immense power through PCTs and care trusts in developing primary care and health improvement strategies for their localities. The 'consultation exercises' carried out by health authorities have a reputation (widespread, if not always justified) of being entirely tokenistic, consisting of the presentation to a hastily assembled public meeting of a decision that has already been taken.

Of all those engaged in developing local health strategies, only local councillors are answerable through the ballot box to the communities affected by them. Some councillors have, indeed, been resistant to the efforts of community workers to encourage a questioning stance by local people. But, whatever their personal inclinations, it is in their interest to ensure that their electorates are genuinely consulted and genuinely satisfied with the outcomes of health improvement initiatives. Local councillors and the authorities they run, having an input into cross-cutting planning, such as regeneration and environmental strategies, are in a position to consult their electorates holistically about all of the issues that affect their lives. In recent years, they have begun to develop imaginative consultation strategies and responses that engage local people in holistic solutions (see, for example, Campbell, 2000, Chapter 6). And there is some indication that health authorities may be recognizing local authority expertise in this area and joining with them in developing corporate consultation strategies across a range of issues (Campbell, 2000, Chapter 5).

Moreover, individual citizens are not neutral about the source of the services they receive. Surveys by local authorities have frequently shown that older people, for example, prefer to live in a local authority run home than in one that is privately run. At the time of writing, an 89-year-old resident of a local authority home is conducting a legal challenge under the Human Rights Act against Birmingham City Council, because the council is planning to transfer its homes to the independent sector. According to her solicitor, most of the 900 residents in Birmingham's homes are opposed to the plans to transfer ownership and 'would prefer to remain in the public sector' (*The Times*, 14 May 2001). Residents of such homes are aware that decisions about their homes and related services are made by people in whose election they have participated and to whom they have local access. They believe that they have rights of ownership in such services that extend well beyond the kind of consumer rights in a commercial relationship that derive from ability to pay. That is why current trends (such as privatization, 'externalization' and 'outsourcing') in both local government and the health service that distance service providers from direct accountability to the electorate are not mere matters of efficiency. There are fundamental issues at stake about the nature of democracy and citizenship.

The close relationship between democratically elected local representatives and the communities they serve is being undermined, not only by privatization, but also by the proliferation of appointed public bodies – 'quangos' –which include health authorities, PCTs, health action zones and health and care trusts (Skelcher et al., 2000). Such quangos are not accountable to local citizens but, in the case of health care, only upwards at best, to a remote secretary of state. There is almost no public access to the decision-making processes of such bodies, and yet in the health arena they are taking decisions to spend public money and increasingly handing it over to the private sector (for example, through the Private Finance Initiative) in ways that will impact on the quality of life of local communities for years to come.

It is true that health quangos are, at least in principle, among the more open and representative members of the 'quango state' (many Health Action Zone boards, for example, publish newsletters about their activities). But even these bodies have nothing like the accountability framework and strict consultation regimes to which local government is answerable. How many of them publish the private addresses and telephone numbers of their board members, as local councils do? How many publish agendas and papers in advance, permit the public to attend and speak at meetings and publish minutes of decisions, as local government is required to do?

The future for local government and its engagement with health improvement is not, therefore, just about recognizing the vast range of its functions that affect people's health. It is also about the processes by which health outcomes are determined. Indeed, the processes can influence the outcomes, and in that sense, democracy is not just an optional extra, but an essential tool for promoting health. Perhaps the new local government power of scrutiny of health services will do something to redress the balance which has been shifting dangerously far from local democratic accountability.

WHAT SHOULD BE THE HEALTH PROMOTION ROLE OF LOCAL GOVERNMENT?

A socio-economic understanding of health presents an apparent dilemma for local authorities. A concentration on the root causes of ill health and inequalities in health suggests that national economic and redistributive policies (for example, through the tax and benefits systems) are most likely to have an impact on health (Davey Smith and Gordon, 2000; Shaw et al., 1999). If such causes are given their due weight, it might seem that there is little for local government to do since it is not in a position to redistribute wealth from one area of the country to another or to make policies on tax and benefits.

Nonetheless, there remains an important space for action between national policy and personal behaviour, in which local government can have a profound effect. In their own geographical regions, local authorities raise taxation (and can use it for redistribution purposes within their own areas) and spend a significant proportion of money raised through national taxation. Many of the services they provide (education, housing, environment, transport and so on) have a direct impact on community health. There are inequalities within communities, as well as between them, and there are local economies as well as a national one – facts that regeneration, anti-poverty and equalities strategies are designed to address. 'Postcode prescribing' is iniquitous when it means that two people in similar circumstances in different parts of the country have different entitlements to treatment. But there is a sense in which postcode prescribing is necessary to enable provision to respond to the different socio-economic circumstances experienced by different groups. In fact, a benign version of postcode prescribing is precisely what local authorities administer when they address inequalities of gender, race and class within their electorates.

But does this simply amount to the fact that local authorities' work will affect health, even if it is not specifically designed to do so? Is there any need for local authorities to address themselves explicitly to health matters, since their work will have an impact in any case? This argument may appear obviously wrong, but it is worth being clear as to why it is wrong.

To take housing as an example, while all local authority housing policies will have an impact on health, some will have an adverse impact (such as the extensive use of temporary bed and breakfast accommodation) while others will have a favourable impact (such as those that provide for the education needs of minorities, access to sources of employment, public transport, affordable nutritional food and primary healthcare, an approach now being adopted in Health Action Zone areas, for example). If improved health is not an *explicit* goal of housing policy, and if housing policies have no understanding of how homelessness and housing impact on health, the policy is less likely to have positive health outcomes than if it has a health dimension built in from the start. Similarly, a broad and inclusive corporate approach to environmental health that looks at issues of pollution and air quality, for example, and avoids the narrow medical model favoured by some environmental health officers, is likely to impact on council policies well beyond a narrowly defined environmental health function.

Furthermore, local authorities can make a genuine contribution to the implementation of national economic policies that impact on health, for example in how they use national funding for regeneration projects, and small local projects can facilitate national redistributive policies. For instance, there is evidence that local authority initiatives to provide benefits take-up advice to deprived communities in locations such as health centres can have a direct effect on individuals' health (Abbott and Hobby, 2000).

This sort of evidence, derived from careful evaluation of focused local initiatives, can act as a driver for change at national level. It is important that local authorities and health partnerships have sufficient flexibility to innovate. In responding to the health needs and aspirations of communities, local government with its health partners can contribute to the development of evidence-based health promotion and prevention strategies by national government. To be 'health blind' in developing policies in areas that impact on health is just as dangerous as to be 'gender blind' in developing policies that impact on gender. That is one good reason for local authorities to develop health impact assessment and health inequalities impact assessment tools that are routinely used at the planning, implementation and evaluation stages of all their polices.

CONCLUSION

Current government policies mean that the role of the local state in relation to health is, in some respects, under siege from both the private sector and the health sector. Despite this, there are some excellent examples of imaginative collaboration between health and local authorities at local level. A progressive vision of public health promotion must continue to recognize the essential contribution of local government.

Health is a complex issue that cuts across different specialist services provided to the public. Local authorities – which provide many such services – are better placed to understand their collective impact on health than any single specialist provider. Furthermore, they have a general duty to plan and power to look to the well-being of their communities, a power which no other body possesses. The best local government would take explicit account of health impact in all its strategic planning. In its ideal form, it could be the locus for all those aspects of democracy that empower individuals as citizens and thereby contribute to their overall health and well-being. It could also be a source of the kind of rights enjoyed by citizens who are more than mere consumers of services.

Perhaps because of the wide range of services it offers, local government is well placed to see local communities in the round and individual citizens as full human beings, as active agents rather than as passive patients. It can and should be (but has not always been) a champion of a social model of health that recognizes the socio-economic determinants of ill health and health inequalities. In this respect, it is in a strong position to support, and lobby for, a progressive approach to public health promotion both locally and nationally.

6.3

CITIZENS ADVICE BUREAUX IN PRIMARY CARE: A TOOL FOR STAFF TO ADDRESS SOCIAL AND ECONOMIC INEQUALITIES

Judith Emanuel

Increasingly, primary care is becoming the focal point for health services in the UK. A major function of the primary care trusts created in 2001 is responsibility for improving the health of their populations and addressing health inequalities; but primary care trusts may be at a loss to know how to tackle these functions, particularly given other pressures. One way of addressing poverty and inequity has been the introduction of Citizens Advice Bureaux (CABx) and welfare rights services into primary care settings. This case study considers one particular issue: how the CAB service in one primary care setting has been an important enabling mechanism for staff who want to address inequalities in health in primary care, but do not always feel they have the resources to do so.

THE STUDY SETTING

The study took place in a primary care practice serving a population of over 12,000 people in Tipton, a small town in the West Midlands, which has high levels of social and economic deprivation and ill health. The practice had over 30 staff, including six GPs and had had a CAB adviser since 1992, when the local health authority started funding CAB services in primary care as part of its regeneration and anti-poverty initiatives (Sandwell Health Authority, 1996).

This case study is based on 20 semi-structured interviews with primary care staff and CAB service users at the practice which was part of a wider study (Emanuel and Begum, 2000). The qualities of the collaboration between CAB and practice staff are explored in an attempt to draw out the important issues.

THE CASE FOR BENEFITS ADVICE IN PRIMARY CARE

Encouraging uptake of state benefits was a recommendation of the *Independent Inquiry into Inequalities in Health* (Acheson, 1998). Over a ten-month period, the CAB adviser saw 603 people with a new problem. Some had more than one problem, so 856 problems were identified, of which 76 per cent related to benefits (Emanuel and Begum, 2000).

Studies which have examined money raised through CAB and welfare rights services in primary care have shown that they can help people to obtain substantial financial benefits to which they are entitled (Paris and Player, 1993; Coppell et al., 1999). In one study, 39 of 150 attendees were eligible for payments totalling over £58,000 in that year, of which nearly £55,000 was recurring (Paris and Player, 1993). Our study (Emanuel and Begum, 2000) suggested that health status improved nine months after referral to the CAB, although these results did not reach statistical significance. However, taken alongside other evidence (Abbott and Hobby, 1999), it seems that health improvement as well as economic benefit can result from CAB services in primary care.

Welfare rights agencies and CABx usually offer a range of services, as well as benefits advice, which vary in different agencies and places. There has been little research on the effectiveness of advice other than benefit advice, because it is harder to measure, or on the advantages and disadvantages of different service providers.

THE CASE STUDY

Our interviewees included the CAB adviser, administrative staff, nurses and doctors, who had worked at the practice for between 15 months and 10 years. The users we interviewed had visited the CAB with a new problem.

For a range of reasons, this case study should be viewed as good practice, rather than typical of CAB or welfare rights services in primary care. The CAB adviser was based at the practice half-time, providing a greater presence than other similar services; the service was mainstream funded and had been so for eight years and was therefore established; the practice and CAB showed an unusual level of shared commitment; the adviser worked full-time in primary care settings and therefore had an unusually high level of experience; and the practice prided itself on innovation, and the staff had strong commitment to addressing deprivation. This case study focuses on doctors and nurses because strong working relationships developed in this practice between the CAB adviser and these two groups.

ENABLING STAFF TO ADDRESS SOCIAL AND ECONOMIC DEPRIVATION

There may be two reasons why it is difficult to address social and economic issues in primary care: first, clinicians may not see it as their role to do this; and, second, clinicians may want to address these issues but do not feel that they have the knowledge, skills or resources needed.

Here, we focus on how CAB involvement enabled motivated clinicians to address inequality. Arblaster and Hastings (2000), in their excellent contribution to the debate, acknowledge the role of the primary carer as 'networker' and Mercer and Barnes (2000) talk similarly about the GP's role as 'gatekeeper'.

CAB services allow the primary care team to extend access to services beyond those traditionally accessed.

Before working with a CAB adviser in the practice, some staff had attempted to respond to social and economic needs but had found it time-consuming or difficult. One nurse acknowledged that, without the resources to deal with these issues, she felt 'a block on that part of the patient'. With the CAB service present, staff felt able to explore a wider set of issues with patients. For example, one nurse said she routinely asked about housing when she saw a patient with asthma, and referred people to the CAB adviser if there was a problem.

HEALTHCARE WORKERS' ROLES IN RELATION TO THE CAB SERVICE

Several of the clinical staff said that having a CAB adviser at the practice extended their awareness of and ability to address the social and economic needs of patients. For example, previously they were likely to accept the outcome of benefit applications but over time they became more aware of the possibilities of appealing against refusals. One clinician said that having the service had made her more aware that filling in forms was a problem for some patients, and that many lacked friends or family who could help with this.

Plans by the CAB adviser and primary care staff to develop a preventive service were also developed. They proposed to target groups within the population served, whether or not a problem had been identified. Groups under consideration included users of community nursing services, people booked in for elective surgery, or people admitted to hospital as an emergency. Primary care staff felt that this broadened their understanding of what the CAB could offer, illustrating that this was a continuing process.

CAB ADVISER AS A MEMBER OF THE PRIMARY HEALTH CARE TEAM

Over time it became clear that the CAB adviser had come to be regarded as a full member of the primary health care team. For example, there was an acceptance by staff that he should have access to confidential patient information in the same way as other members of the team. There was also evidence of collaborative work with team members about individual patients, as well as about service development. The CAB adviser consulted clinical colleagues about users' medical problems, while health workers consulted the adviser about social or economic problems. 'Because he might want to come and say . . . what do you really think about them (the patient)? And (we) work it (a benefit application or appeal) up together . . . which I guess would not happen if he were based off site.'

The adviser also attended the weekly nurses' meeting, where individual patients might be discussed as well as service developments. His participation illustrated active teamwork, as described by one of the nurses: 'well for him to be readily there if something comes to mind and perhaps for him to pick up on when we are talking about the patients, he might pick up himself that perhaps they might need . . . I could get involved and visit.'

Workload

Clinical staff felt that having a CAB adviser in the practice improved patient care, rather than reducing their workload. Where they had to write more reports, they valued the advice of the CAB adviser about what they should cover.

Moffatt et al. (1999) found that primary health care staff thought that addressing financial and material aspects of patients' welfare would increase workload, while Abbott and Hobby (1999) discussed GPs' anxieties about extra and unrewarded work. This issue of the relationship between workload and addressing the social and economic needs of primary care users is an important one to address if primary care staff are to take a broader role.

One member of staff sometimes found patients told her things she found very worrying, but lacked any staff counselling service she might turn to. She said having an agency to pass such problems on to 'offloaded some of that emotional worry', suggesting that having a CAB service might enable staff to address issues that would otherwise impose an intolerable strain.

THE CAB APPROACH

The CAB adviser concentrated not only on the quality of advice he gave, but also on the process of giving advice. This way of working might give staff access to skills which had not featured in their own training. The way in which help was offered was particularly important for some interviewees, especially those who had been in anxious or nervous states when they first saw the CAB adviser. An interviewee said that he was nervous, anxious and irritable on his first visit, but described how over time the adviser had skilfully made the interviewee comfortable so that sessions moved from being 'monologue to dialogue'.

After having all the information to consider, two interviewees decided that they did not want to pursue an application or an appeal. As one put it: 'He guides you but doesn't tell you what to do.' This related closely to the intention of the CAB adviser, who saw his role as presenting options, but not to make decisions for people. It was also in line with the overall aim of the CAB service, which is not to solve problems but to enable clients 'to manage their own problems by helping them to use their own skills and abilities' (NACAB, 1998). The adviser felt that, at times, this was difficult because many people find it hard to make decisions. Their problems may be complex and there is time pressure within a 30-minute interview. If they are unable to reach a decision, he will advise them to come back when they have made a decision, which he reported they usually did. He sees that 'the choice of the individual is paramount'. Finally, one interviewee said that it was clear who was responsible for what: 'He sat down and talked you through a situation . . . what he was going to do and what I had to do myself.'

MEDICALIZATION OR HOLISM?

Some health service planners and clinicians argue that it is unnecessary for this type of service to be based in the practice, instead, clinicians should refer to outside agencies. They are concerned that by integrating non-medical services into a primary care setting, issues such as benefits will be increasingly 'medicalized'. By contrast, others feel that a holistic service demands this range of services in the health care setting (Emanuel, 1998).

It was clear that having the CAB adviser based in the building was crucial to this practice, for a range of reasons. Most staff were not familiar with the CAB prior to this involvement, so working with the adviser led to new understanding of what the CAB could offer. Many staff preferred this kind of learning to formal training. Their knowledge also developed over time; some reported that they had initially referred only benefit problems but that the range they referred had broadened over time. It might be argued that joint working does not depend on a shared base. But although the primary care staff trusted the CAB adviser in the practice, this trust did not extend to the CAB as a whole.

It was apparent that staff believed that having the adviser based in the practice was crucial to the development of joint working and had enabled them to adopt a more holistic approach to their patients. For example, one GP found the service particularly useful for people who needed to leave work for medical reasons, especially if they were not in a trade union, so that they could weigh up the financial implications. The GP was aware that if they lost out financially they could end up in a worse situation. She recognised that the service could be used proactively, and that medical needs had to be weighed up against social and economic needs, which could conflict.

Moffatt et al. (1999) have suggested that such services may work best if they are seen by staff as an appropriate health care intervention. This appears to have been crucial to the successful integration of the CAB into the services offered by this practice and staff believed that having the adviser based in the practice was essential to this success.

CONCLUSION

Primary care trusts have an obligation to address inequalities in health. This case study shows why even primary health care workers who want to do this may find it difficult to integrate into their routine practice, and indicates how the introduction of a CAB service can help to overcome some of the obstacles.

The work reported here builds on a developing body of evidence that provision of CAB and welfare rights advice is an effective way to improve uptake of benefits, and leads to substantial financial benefits for practice populations and to improvements in health status for those who gain such benefits. It is not only the service itself that is important, but also how it is integrated in primary care. This case study is transferable to other primary care settings and, with the development of primary care trusts, the opportunities for the introduction of CAB and welfare rights initiatives like this will, hopefully, increase.

ACKNOWLEDGEMENTS

Many thanks to Stephen Abbott, Liz Jayne and the editors of the book for their constructive comments on the first draft of this case study.

CONCLUSION

What are the biggest threats to health we face? While much effort by health promoters and public health specialists is directed at trying to change 'lifestyles' or prevent particular diseases or their complications, there are bigger issues at stake. It is not just that health is 'more than the absence of disease', but that a prerequisite for both health and disease is our survival – and ensuring that will be one of the greatest challenges of the coming century. We believe that the major and persisting threats to health, in our 'modern' world, are human conflict, environmental degradation, increasing political and material inequality within and between nations, and the marketization or privatization of public services. In the face of such challenges, public health strategies which are disease- or behaviour-focused will no longer do the trick – if they ever did.

The Health For All declaration has long noted that peace is a prerequisite for health. Despite so many images and reports over the past decade from the 'trouble spots' of the world – the Middle East, the Balkans, South East Asia, even Northern Ireland – and the involvement of our own governments in many of these conflicts, it still seems too easy to forget this fundamental point. The necessity for peace should at least remind us, had we forgotten, of the close relationship between politics and health.

The survival of our fragile eco-system will also be a pressing concern for the century ahead. Human activity – much of it transnational corporate activity – is already causing global climate change. We can expect an increased frequency of severe weather events, rising sea levels, changed food growing conditions, spreading insect-borne diseases and mass migration of populations. In addition, the continuing economic concentration of such 'industries' as farming leads to immediate environmental costs through the increasing use of heavy freight transport to move goods long distances, increasing congestion and the demand for yet more roads. Everywhere that environmental damage and upheaval occur, whether the result of global forces or of local economic activity, the poorest will suffer first and most directly, while the better off try – but will ultimately fail – to avoid the impact. It is clear that environmental justice, alongside social justice, must now become a strong demand for public health promoters.

The widening income inequality of the past two decades, especially in the UK and the USA, has rightly become a focus for research and policy debate by many concerned about public health. As has been noted throughout this book, increasing material inequality threatens not only the health of the poor, but the health of all, and is also associated with crime and social unrest within countries, and migration between them. Yet we are also seeing growing inequality in political power in the UK, with centralization of government control over public services, erosion of local democratic accountability, the 'quangoization' of the state, and the increasing influence of profit-making corporate interests in many areas of public life. Meanwhile, internationally the growth of corporate power means that many nations – even developed nations – find themselves trading with companies economically bigger and more powerful than they are.

In such a global context, it is no surprise to find many governments, including the UK government, encouraging an increasing role for unaccountable, commercial organizations in both the provision and financing of public services. The health arguments not simply for public services such as health care, education and transport, but also for their public ownership, have been discussed earlier in this book. Once privatized, services – such as the rail network – are difficult to take back into public ownership, even in the presence of strong public support. Despite the lack of evidence of any benefit following from the market reforms of the health service in 1991, or of the supposed greater efficiency of private hospitals over their public counterparts, current policy supports a continued gradual shift of ownership of hospitals and primary care facilities to the private sector together with pressure to make greater use of for-profit providers in many areas of care, such as elective surgery and long-term care.

If these are the most potent challenges to health, what are the greatest obstacles to those working, locally or nationally, for health improvement? The first is the generally unsupportive, or even hostile, policy climate for health. Too often, health is seen as a luxury which should only be considered after other, 'more important' objectives have been assured, such as attracting inward investment locally or increasing GDP nationally. Health is a 'soft', unmeasurable benefit which must come second to hard outcomes such as economic growth, turnover or service delivery. Assessing the health impact of social or economic regeneration schemes may be seen as an obstacle, rather than the whole point of the activity. Even within the health service, which is where the majority of public health promotion professionals work, the idea of public health is poorly understood, with doctors still thinking in terms of preventing infections and managers in terms of meeting coronary heart disease targets. The idea of improving health through democracy, participation, equality or accountability is barely grasped.

One related issue is that of professional division and isolation. Different understandings of health and how to promote it have resulted in competing and sometimes mutually suspicious professional groups who expend much effort in taking up self-justificatory postures. At the same time, there are many other groups of workers – often in local authority settings – who understand that the work they do, for example in housing, town planning, or consumer protection, has health implications but they lack expertise or access to advice on integrating a health dimension into their work. A strong, coherent and broad-based body of professionals is required who are available to national, regional and local policy-makers and service providers – and also to the communities they serve – and who can advise on the health implications of policy issues and help in taking practical action for health.

Such thoughts raise questions about what public health promotion is, and could be. As neither policy-makers nor direct service providers, health promoters of all kinds tend to sit uncomfortably between these poles, nudging the machinery of the local state and local services in the direction of a more positive health impact. This position seems inherently ambiguous, lacking in formal power or authority but working, at best, through influence, advice and persuasion. It is both 'in and against' the state. The continuing, largely theoretical, debate about the independence of the annual reports of directors of public health demonstrates the political tensions which inevitably result from such a position. Although improving health will remain a political project with the tensions and conflicts that entails, the current marginal position of the public health agenda in the NHS and local authorities is by no means inevitable. It is possible to imagine organizations in which, for example, public health equity is taken seriously as a central task, and audited as rigorously and as regularly as the financial position. But for this to occur, the health of communities and populations would have to be high profile issues at national and local level, and of course this is currently not the case.

The ambiguity in the nature of public health promotion is also apparent in the debate over the role of 'evidence' in improving health. Local people with concerns over health issues, for example, the dangers of waste dumping, industrial emissions or traffic volumes, often find themselves ignored because public authorities are reluctant to act in the absence of any evidence that health is being harmed. Similarly, health promoters face difficulties in justifying approaches such as community development without evidence of the 'effectiveness' of their methods. Often, public authorities will make the crude judgement that the lack of any evidence of effect is simply the same as evidence of a lack of effect. Even where evidence is available, it frequently proves to be the 'wrong type' – occupying a different evidential paradigm to that of the decision-maker – and is unable to support the argument either way. If promoting health is primarily a technical task, then of course robust, good quality evidence seems to be essential. However, many of the changes argued for in this book are primarily about the distribution of power and resources, rather than about particular technical interventions. To the extent that these are seen as simply the means to the end of better health, then it is reasonable to demand evidence to support them. But if, for example, local democracy, public accountability, a clean and pleasant environment or accessible services are seen as good in themselves, as worth having even without any consequent measurable health benefits, then the need for evidence is much less obvious.

In this book, many authors have described the importance of local strategies and projects to promote health and reduce inequality in very practical ways. From anti-poverty projects to food co-operatives, and from benefits advice to community development projects, there is clearly much scope for action which can bring real improvements to the lives of local people and can also help to highlight local needs which would otherwise remain invisible. There remains a question, however, over how far such local action can ultimately overcome, rather than simply ameliorate, the major threats to health which we have discussed above.

Can local action ever lead to structural changes which reduce threats to health? By themselves, local projects will produce only local effects, but shared more widely they may inspire others to do something similar – and many people doing similar things in their own localities is social change, albeit in a small way. National or international changes in policy require lobbying, either alone or, better, in alliances with others. Despite the very many people involved in health-related initiatives, a strong public health movement has not yet emerged (though the UK Public Health Association may yet fill this role). Although there are very many single issue campaigns which have a clear relevance to public health, for example, on food, air quality, child poverty, housing, transport, and so on, we have lacked a broad-based movement with a clear understanding of how health is enhanced or damaged and which is able to put forward a wide range of demands for specific policies which will improve health. Instead, the pressure for change has very often been left to individual consumers or consumerist lobby groups which have had some notable successes in particular areas, such as GM food retailing. Public health advocates would do well to study the tactics of consumer organizations, community activists and environmentalists, and learn from their successes.

'Consumer consciousness', however, will not help when it comes to securing policies to reduce widening material inequality, protect the ecosystem from further harm or ensure effective and accessible public services. To make progress on the big issues we need to promote a radical vision of a society far more equal, more sustainable and more healthy than our own – and existing public health and health promotion professionals cannot do this in isolation. Far broader alliances – particularly with environmentalists, anti-poverty workers, trade unionists and campaigners for open and accountable government – are needed to create and support such a vision. We hope that, in this book, we have demonstrated that it is both necessary, and possible, for public health promoters to move beyond their traditional ways of working and to engage with others to this end.

BIBLIOGRAPHY

Abbott, S. and Hobby, L. (1999) 'An evaluation of the Health and Advice Project: its impact on the health of those using the service'. *HaCCRU Research Report 99/63*. Liverpool: Health and Community Care Research Unit, University of Liverpool.

Abbott, S. and Hobby, L. (2000) *Impact of Benefits Advice on Health: An Evaluation of the Health and Advice Project*. Liverpool: Health and Community Care Research Unit, University of Liverpool.

Abel Smith, B. and Townsend, P. (1965) *The Poor and the Poorest*. London: G. Bell and Sons.

Acheson, D. (1998) *Independent Inquiry into Inequalities in Health*. London: The Stationery Office.

Adams, L. (1993) *Health Promotion at the Crossroads: A Study of Health Promotion Departments in the Reorganised NHS*. London: Society of Health Promotion and Health Education Specialists.

Adams, L. (1994) 'Health promotion in crisis', *Health Education Journal* 53 (3): 354–60.

Adams, L. and Armstrong, E. (1996) 'Penrith paradoxes: from analysis to synthesis II – the revenge: a report of the symposium', *Health Care Analysis* 4 (2): 112–19.

Adams, L. and Pintus, S. (1994) 'A challenge to prevailing theory and practice', *Critical Public Health* 5 (2): 17–29.

Agyeman, J. and Evans, B. (1996) 'Black on green: race, ethnicity and the environment', in S. Buckingham-Hatfield and B. Evans (eds) *Environmental Planning and Sustainability*, Chichester: Wiley.

Alcock, P. (1997) *Understanding Poverty*, Basingstoke: Macmillan.

Alcock, P. et al. (2000). *Wakefield HAZ Evaluation Report*. Wakefield: Wakefield Health Action Zone.

Alcock, P. et al. (2001) *Wakefield HAZ Evaluation Report*. Wakefield: Wakefield Health Action Zone.

Alcock, P., Craig, G., Dalgliesh, K. and Pearson, S. (1995) *Combating Local Poverty: The Management of Anti-Poverty Strategies by Local Government*. Luton: Local Government Management Board.

Allanou, R., Hansen, B. and van der Bilt, Y. (1999) *Public Availability of Data on EU High Production Volume Chemicals*. Ispra, Italy: European Chemicals Bureau. http://ecb.ei.jrc.it/Data-Availability-Documents/datavail.pdf

Allinsky, S. (1969) *Reveille for radicals*, New York: Vintage.

Allison, K. and Rootman, I. (1996) 'Scientific rigour and community participation in health promotion research: are they compatible?', *Health Promotion International* 11 (4): 333—9.

Ambrose, P. (1996) *I Mustn't Laugh Too Much: Health and Housing on the Limehouse Fields and Ocean Estates in Stepney*. Brighton: Centre for Urban and Regional Research, University of Sussex.

Arblaster, L. and Hastings, A. (2000) 'Socio-economic inequality: beyond the inverse care law', in P. Tovey (ed.) *Contemporary Primary Care: The Challenges of Change*. Buckingham: Open University Press.

Argyris, C. and Schön, D.A. (1974) *Theory in Practice: Increasing Professional Effectiveness*. San Francisco: Jossey-Bass.

Armstrong, D. (1993) 'From clinical gaze to regime of total health', in A. Beattie, L. Jones, M. Gott and M. Sidell (eds) *Health and Wellbeing: A Reader*, Basingstoke: Macmillan.

Armstrong, H. (2000) Speech delivered by Minister for Local Government and the Regions to the New Deal for Communities Conference in Brighton, January 25.

Athanasiou, T. (1996) *Slow Reckoning: The Ecology of a Divided Planet*. London: Secker and Warburg.

Audit Commission (1989) *Urban Regeneration and Economic Development: The Local Government Dimension*. London: HMSO.

Audit Commission (1999) *Safety in Numbers: Promoting Community Safety*. Norwich: The Stationery Office.

Baric, L. (1993) 'The settings approach: implications for policy and strategy' *Journal of the Institute of Health Education*, 31 (1): 17–24.

Barnes, C. (1991) *Disabled People in Britain and Discrimination*. London: Hurst and Co.

Barnes, C. and Mercer, G. (eds) (1997) *Doing Disability Research*. Leeds: The Disability Press.

Barnes, M. (1997) *Care, Communities and Citizens*. Harlow: Addison-Wesley Longman.

Barnes, M. and Bennet, G. (1998) 'Frail bodies, courageous voices: older people influencing community care', *Health and Social Care in the Community* 6 (2): 102–11.

Barnes, M. and Bowl, R. (2001) *Taking Over the Asylum: Empowerment and Mental Health*. Basingstoke: Palgrave.

Barnes, M. and Prior, D. (2000) *Private Lives as Public Policy*, Birmingham: Venture Press.

Barnes, M. and Shardlow, P. (1996) 'Identity crisis? Mental health user groups and the "problem" of identity', in C. Barnes and G. Mercer (eds) *Exploring the Divide: Illness and Disability*. Leeds: The Disability Press.

Barnes, M. and Shaw, S. (2000) 'Older people, citizenship and collective action', in A. Warnes, L. Warren and M. Nolan (eds) *Care Services in Later Life*. London: Jessica Kingsley.

Barnes, M. and Wistow, G. (1994) 'Learning to hear voices: listening to users of mental health services', *Journal of Mental Health* 3: 525–40.

Barr, A. et al. (1996) *Measuring Community Development in Northern Ireland: A Handbook for Practitioners*. Belfast: Department of Health and Social Services.

Bartley, M. (1994) 'Unemployment and ill health: understanding the relationship', *Journal of Epidemiology and Community Health* 48 (4): 333–7.

Bartley, M., Ferrie, J. and Montgomery, S.M. (1999) 'Living in a high-unemployment economy: understanding the health consequences', in M. Marmot and R.G. Wilkinson (eds) *Social Determinants of Health*. Oxford: Oxford University Press.

Baum, F. (1990) 'The new public health: force for change or reaction?', *Health Promotion International* 5 (2): 145–50.

Baum, F. (1998) *The New Public Health: An Australian Perspective*. Melbourne: Oxford University Press.

Beattie, A. (1987) 'Making a curriculum work', in P. Allen and M. Jolley (eds) *The Curriculum in Nursing Education*. London: Croom Helm.

Beattie, A. (1990) *Teaching and Learning about Health Education: New Directions in Curriculum Development*. Edinburgh: Health Education Board for Scotland.

Beattie, A. (1995) 'Evaluation in community development for health: an opportunity for dialogue', *Health Education Journal*, 54: 465–72.

Beattie, A. (1996) 'The health promoting school: from idea to action', in A. Scriven and J. Orme (eds) *Health Promotion: Professional Perspectives*, 1st edn. London: Macmillan.

Beattie, A. (1998) 'Action learning for health on campus', in A. Tsouros, G. Dowding, J. Thompson and M. Dooris (eds) *Health Promoting Universities*. Copenhagen: WHO.

Beattie, A. (2001) 'The health promoting school as a learning organisation', in A. Scriven and J. Orme (eds) *Health Promotion: Professional Perspectives*. 2nd edn. London: Macmillan.

Benzeval, A., Judge, K. and Whitehead, M. (eds) (1995) *Tackling Inequalities in Health: An Agenda for Action,* London: King's Fund.

Beresford, P., Green, D., Lister, R. and Woodward, K. (1999) *Poverty First Hand: Poor People Speak for Themselves*. London: Child Poverty Action Group.

Berthoud, R., Benson, S. and Williams, S. (1986) *Standing up for Claimants: Welfare Rights Work in Local Authorities*. London: Policy Studies Institute.

Bevan, A. (1952) *In Place of Fear*. Reprinted (1990) London: Quartet.

Biffa (1997) *Great Britain plc: The Environmental Balance Sheet*. High Wycombe: Biffa Waste Services.

Bjaras, G., Haglund, B.J.A. and Rifkin, S. (1991) 'A new approach to community participation assessment', *Health Promotion International* 6 (3): 199–206.

Black, M. (1994) *Celebrating Community Development and Health*. Conference report, Belfast: Community Development and Health Network.

Blackman, T. (1995) *Urban Policy in Practice*. London: Routledge.

Blair, D., Giesecke, C.G. and Sherman, S. (1991) 'A dietary, social and economic evaluation of the Philadelphia Urban Gardening Project', *Journal of Nutrition Education*, 23 (4): 161–7.

Blair, T. (2000) Speech to Labour Party conference, September.

Blane, D., Davey Smith, G. and Bartley, M. (1990) 'Social class differences in years of potential life lost: size, trends and principal causes', *BMJ*, 301: 429–32.

Blaxter, M. (1990) *Health and Lifestyles*, London: Tavistock/Routledge.

Bloomfield, K. (1998) *We Will Remember Them: Report of the NI Victims Commissioner*. Belfast: Northern Ireland Office.

Blowers, A. (1997) 'Environmental policy: ecological modernisation or the risk society?' *Urban Studies*, 34 (5–6): 845–71.

Boardman, B., Bullock, S. and McLaren, D. (1999) *Equity and the Environment: Guidelines for Green and Socially Just Government*. London: Catalyst/Friends of the Earth.

Bracht, N. (ed.) (1999) *Health Promotion at the Community Level: New Advances*. 2nd edn. Thousand Oaks, CA: Sage.

Bradshaw, J. (1975) 'Welfare rights: an experimental approach', in R. Lees and G. Smith (eds) *Action Research in Community Development*. London: Routledge and Kegan Paul.

Brannen, J., Dodd, K., Oakley, A. and Storey, P. (1994) *Young People, Health and Family Life*. Buckingham: Open University Press.

Brazier, J.E., Harper, R., Jones, N.M.B., O'Cathain, A., Thomas, K.J., Usherwood, T. and Westlake, L. (1992) 'Validating the SF-36 health survey questionnaire: a new outcome measure for primary care', *BMJ*, 305: 160–4.

Brehm, J. and Rahn, W. (1997) 'Individual level evidence for the causes and consequences of social capital', *American Journal of Political Science*, 41: 999–1023.

Brookfield, S. (1983) 'Adult learning groups, community development and community action', Chapter 5 in *Adult Learners, Adult Education and the Community*. Buckingham: Open University Press.

Brunner, E. and Marmot, M. (1999) 'Social organization, stress and health', in M.G. Marmot and R.G. Wilkinson (eds) *The Social Determinants of Health*. Oxford: Oxford University Press.

Bullard, R. (1993) 'Anatomy of environmental racism and the environmental justice movement', in R.D. Bullard (ed.) *Confronting Environmental Racism: Voices from the Grassroots*. Boston: South End Press.

Bullock, S. (1995) *Prescription for Change*. London: Friends of the Earth.

Bulmer, M. (1987) *The Social Basis of Community Care*. London: Allen and Unwin.

Bunker, J.P., Frazier, H.S. and Mosteller, F. (1994) 'Improving health: measuring effects of medical care', *Millbank Quarterly*, 72: 225–58.

Bunton, R. (1992) 'More than a woolly jumper: health promotion as social regulation', *Critical Public Health*, 3 (2): 4–11.

Cabinet Office (2000) *Strategy for neighbourhood renewal*, at: http://www.cabinet-office.gov.uk/seu/2000/Nat_Strat_Cons/contents.htm

Calder, J. (1984) 'The Open University's health education programme', in R. Lewis (ed.) *Open Learning in Action*. London: CET.

Calhoun, C. (ed.) (1997) *Habermas and the Public Sphere*. Cambridge, MA: MIT Press.

Calman, K.C. (1998) *The Potential for Health*. Oxford: Oxford University Press.

Cambridge Econometrics (1998) *Industrial benefits from environmental tax reform in the UK*. Cambridge: Cambridge Econometrics.

Campbell, C. et al. (1998) *Developing Social Indicators for Health Promotion: Exploratory Research into the Role of Social Capital*. London: Health Education Authority.

Campbell, C., Wood, R. and Kelly, M. (1999) *Social Capital and Health*. London: Health Education Authority.

Campbell, F. (ed.) (2000) *Building Healthy Communities: The Role of Local Government in Health Improvement*. London: Local Government Information Unit.

Campbell, J. and Oliver, M. (1996) *Disability Politics: Understanding our Past, Changing our Future*. London: Routledge.

Capek, S.M. (1993) 'The "environmental justice" frame: a conceptual discussion and an application', *Social Problems*, 40 (1): 5–22.

Caraher, M., Dixon, P., Lang, T. and Carr-Hill, R. (1998) 'Barriers to accessing healthy foods: differentials by gender, social class, income and mode of transport,' *Health Education Journal*, 57 (3), 191–201.

Carley, M. and Spapens, P. (1998) *Sharing the World*. London: Earthscan.

Chadwick, E. (1842) *The Report on the Sanitary Condition of the Labouring Population of Great Britain*. Reprinted M.W. Flynn (ed.) (1979) Edinburgh: Edinburgh University Press.

Charles, N. and Kerr, M. (1986) 'Issues of responsibility and control in the feeding of families', in S. Rodmell and A. Watt, (eds) *The Politics of Health Education: Raising the Issues*. London: Routledge and Kegan Paul.

Chartered Institute of Environmental Health (CIEH) (1999) *Health Promotion Policy*. At: http://www.cieh.org.uk/about/policy/policy/healthpolicy.htm.

Chief Medical Officer (1999) *The Health of the Public in Northern Ireland: Report of the Chief Medical Officer*. Belfast: Northern Ireland Department of Health and Social Services.

Chitty, C. and Simon, B. (eds) (1994) *Education Answers Back: Critical Responses to Government Policy*. London: Lawrence & Wishart.

Clunies-Ross, T. and Hildyard, N. (1992) *The Politics of Industrial Agriculture*. London: Earthscan.

Cobb, S. and Kasl, S.C. (1977) *Termination: The Consequence of Job Loss*. Cincinnati: Department of Health, Education and Welfare. Publication no 77–224. US National Institutes for Occupational Safety and Health.

Coburn, D. (2000) 'Income inequality, social cohesion and the health status of populations: the role of neo- liberalism', *Social Science and Medicine* 51: 135–46.

Cohen, J.L. (1985) 'Strategy or identity: new theoretical paradigms and contemporary social movements', *Social Research*, 52 (4): 663–716.

Cohen, J.L. and Arato, A. (1992) *Civil Society and Political Theory*. Cambridge, MA: MIT Press.

Coleman, J.S. (1988) 'Social capital in the creation of human capital', *American Journal of Sociology*, Supplement: S95–S120.

Community Development Project (1977) *Gilding the Ghetto: the State and the Poverty Experiments*. Coventry: CDP.

Cooper, H., Arber, S., Fee, L. and Ginn, J. (1999) *The Influence of Social Support and Social Capital on Health: A Review of British Data*. London: Health Education Authority.

Coppell, D.H., Packham, C.J. and Varnam, M.A. (1999) 'Providing welfare rights in primary care', *Public Health*, 113: 131–5.

Cormie, J. (1999) 'The Fife User Panels Project: empowering older people', in M. Barnes and L. Warren (eds) *Paths to Empowerment*. Bristol: The Policy Press.

Cornwell, J. (1984) *Hard-earned Lives*. London: Tavistock.

Craig, G. (1989) 'Community work and the state', *Community Development Journal*, 24 (1): 3–18.

Craig, G. and Mayo, M. (eds) (1994) *Community Empowerment: A Reader in Participation and Development*. London: Zed Books.

Crewe, F.A.E. (1945) *Social Medicine: An Academic Discipline and an Instrument of Social Policy*. Edinburgh: Graduates' Association.

Crotty, P. (1999) 'Food and class', in J. Germov and L. Williams (eds) *A Sociology of Food and Nutrition: The Social Appetite*. Melbourne: Oxford University Press.

Culyer, A.J. (1976) *Need and the National Health Service: Economics and Social Choice*. Oxford: Martin Robertson.

Dahlberg, K. (1992) *Report and Recommendations on the Knoxville, Tennessee, Food System*. Kalamazoo: Western Michigan University.

Dahlgren, G. and Whitehead, M. (1991) *Policies and Strategies to Promote Equity in Health*. Stockholm: Institute for Futures Studies (mimeo).

Davey, B. (1999) 'Solving economic, social and environmental problems together: an empowerment strategy for losers' in M. Barnes and L. Warren (eds) *Paths to Empowerment*. Bristol: The Policy Press.

Davey Smith, G. (1996) 'Income inequality and mortality and why they are related', *BMJ*, 20 April: 987–8.

Davey Smith, G. and Gordon, D. (2000) 'Poverty across the life course and health', in C. Pantazis and D. Gordon (eds) *Tackling Inequalities: Where We Are Now and What Can Be Done?* Bristol: Policy Press.

Davis, K. (1993) 'On the movement', in J. Swain et al. *Disabling Barriers: Enabling Environments*. London: Sage.

Deakin, N. and Edwards, J. (1993) *The Enterprise Culture and the Inner City*. London: Routledge.

Department for Education and Employment (1998) *Employment of Disabled People*. London: DEE.

Department of Health (1992) *Health of the Nation*. London: Department of Health.

Department of Health (1996) *Women's Health Promotion: A Resource Pack for Health Care Purchasers and Providers*. London: Department of Health.

Department of Health (1997) *The New NHS – Modern, Dependable*. London: The Stationery Office.

Department of Health (1998) *Our Healthier Nation: A Contract for Health*. London: The Stationery Office.

Department of Health (1999a) *Reducing Health Inequalities: An Action Report*. London: Department of Health.

Department of Health (1999b) *Saving Lives: Our Healthier Nation*. London: Department of Health.

Department of Health (2000a) *Coronary Heart Disease National Service Framework*. London: Department of Health.

Department of Health (2000b) *For the Benefit of Patients: A Concordat with the Private and Voluntary Health Care Provider Sector*. London: Department of Health.

Department of Health (2000c) *Policy Action Team 13*. http://www.doh.gov.uk/shoppingaccess.htm.

Department of Health, Health and Social Care Joint Unit (2001) *Care Trusts: Emerging Framework*. London: Department of Health.

Department of Health and Social Security (1980) *Inequalities in Health: Report of a Research Group*. London: DHSS.

Department of Social Security (1999) *Opportunity for All: Tackling Poverty and Social Exclusion*. London: Stationery Office.

DETR (1997) *Regeneration Programmes – The Way Forward*. London: The Stationery Office.

DETR (1999a) *The Air Quality Strategy for England, Wales, and Northern Ireland*. London: Department for Environment, Transport and the Regions.

DETR (1999b) *A Better Quality of Life: A Strategy for Sustainable Development in the UK*. London: The Stationery Office: http://www.environment.detr.gov.uk/sustainable/quality/life/index.htm

DETR (2000a) *Guidance on Community Planning*. Norwich: The Stationery Office.

DETR (2000b) *Guidance on the Preparation of Regional Sustainable Development Frameworks*. London: Department for Environment, Transport and the Regions.

DETR (2000c) *Local Government Research Summary: Cross-Cutting Issues in Public Policy and Public Service*. London: Department for Environment, Transport and the Regions.

DETR (2000d) *Preparing Community Strategies: Draft Guidance to Local Authorities*. London: DETR.

DHSS (1996) *Health and Wellbeing – into the Next Millennium: Regional Strategy for Health 1997–2002*. Belfast: Northern Ireland Department of Health and Social Services.

DHSS (1997a) *Targeting Health and Social Need: The Contribution of Nursing*. Belfast: Northern Ireland Department of Health and Social Services.

DHSS (1997b) *Well in 2000*. Belfast: Northern Ireland Department of Health and Social Services.

DHSS Voluntary Activity Unit (1999) *Mainstreaming Community Development in the Personal Health and Social Services*. Belfast: Northern Ireland Department of Health and Social Services.

Dobson, B. (1997) 'The paradox of want amidst plenty: from food poverty to social exclusion', in N.M. Köhler, E. Feichtinger, E. Barlösius and E. Dowler (eds) *Poverty and Food in Welfare Societies*. Berlin: WZB.

Dobson, B., Beardsworth, A., Keil, T. and Walker, R. (1994) *Diet, Choice and Poverty: Social, Cultural and Nutritional Aspects of Food Consumption Among Low Income Families.* Loughborough: Loughborough University of Technology, Centre for Research in Social Policy.

Dolk, H., Vrijheid, M., Armstrong, B., Abramsky, L., Bianchi, F., Garne, E., Nelen, V., Robert, E., Scott, J.E.S., Stone, D. and Tenconi, R. (1998) 'Risk of congenital anomalies near hazardous-waste landfill sites in Europe: the EUROHAZCON study,' *Lancet* 352: 423–7.

Donne, J. (1624) *Devotions upon Emergent Occasions.* London.

Dowler, E. (1998) 'Food poverty and food policy', *IDS bulletin. Poverty and Social Exclusion in North and South*, 29 (1): 58–65.

Dowler, E. (1999) 'Food and poverty: the present challenge', *Benefits*, 24: 3–6.

Dowling, S. (1983) *Health for a Change: The Provision of Preventive Health Care in Pregnancy and Early Childhood.* London: Child Poverty Action Group.

Doyal, L. (1995) *What Makes Women Sick: Gender and the Political Economy of Health,* Basingstoke: Macmillan.

Draper, P. (ed.) (1991) *Health through Public Policy: The Greening of Public Health,* London: Green Print.

Drewnoski, A. and Popkin, K. (1997) 'The nutrition transition: new trends in the global diet'. *Nutrition Reviews*, 55, 31–43.

Driedger, D. (1989) *The Last Civil Rights Movement.* London: Hurst and Co.

Duckett, S. (2001) 'Does it matter who owns health facilities?', *Journal of Health Services Research and Policy*, 6 (1): 59–62.

Duffy, T.M. and Cunningham, D.J. (1996) 'Constructivism: implications for the design and delivery of instruction', in D.H. Jonassen (ed.) *Handbook of Research for Educational Communications and Technology.* New York: Simon & Schuster.

Duncan, P. and Thomas, S. (2000) *Neighbourhood Regeneration: Resourcing Community Involvement.* Bristol: The Policy Press.

Dunne, M.C. (1993) *Stitched Up: Action for Health in Ancoats, Voices of Struggle, Hope and Vision.* Manchester: Church Action on Poverty.

East End Quality of Life (2000a) *Tinsley Community Health and Transport Project: Final Report and Evaluation.* Sheffield: East End Quality of Life Project.

East End Quality of Life (2000b) *Health Impact Assessment on the Rotherham and Sheffield M1 Motorway Corridor Planning Study.* Sheffield: East End Quality of Life Project.

Emanuel, J. (1998) *Citizens Advice Bureaux in General Practice. Report 1: Commissioning.* Manchester: Centre for Public Health and Health Promotion, University of Manchester.

Emanuel, J. and Begum, S. (2000) *What Do you Advise, Doc? A Citizen's Advice Bureau in Primary Care in the West Midlands.* Manchester: Centre for Higher and Adult Education, University of Manchester.

Employment Policy Institute (1999) *Economic Report: The Environment.* 14 (1): 1–23. London: Employment Policy Institute.

ENDS (1998a) 'Inconsistent regulation pushes polluted soil into Scotland', *The ENDS Report*, 277: 14–15. London: Environmental Data Services.

ENDS (1998b) 'Scotland's feeble fines for industrial pollution', *The ENDS Report*, 285: 51. London: Environmental Data Services.

ENDS (1999) 'Prosecution rate, fines remain at low level in Scotland', *The ENDS Report*, 295: 51. London: Environmental Data Services.

Engels, F. (1973) *The Condition of the Working Class in England*. Moscow: Progress Publishers.

Equal Ability (1999) *Disabiling Practice and How to Avoid It*. Horbury: Equal Ability.

Etzioni, A. (1995) *The Spirit of Community*. London: Collins.

FAO (1999) *Food Insecurity: When People Must Live with Hunger and Fear of Starvation*. Rome: Food and Agriculture Organisation.

FAO/WHO (1992) *International Conference on Nutrition*. Rome: Food and Agriculture Organisation.

Faulkner, A. and Layzell, S. (2000) *Strategies for Living: A Report of User Led Research into People's Strategies for Living with Mental Distress*. London: Mental Health Foundation.

Feuerstein, M.T. (1988) 'Finding the methods to fit the people: training for participatory evaluation', *Community Development Journal*, 23: 16–25.

Fine, B. (1993) 'Resolving the diet paradox', *Social Science and Information*, 32(4) 669–87.

Finkelstein, V. and Stuart, O. (1996) 'Developing new services', in G. Hales (ed.) *Beyond Disability: Towards an Enabling Society*. London: Sage: 170–87.

Foodworks Enquiry (1997) *From Food Deserts to Food Security; An Alternative Vision*. Glasgow: The Poverty Alliance.

Freire, P. (1972) *Pedagogy of the Oppressed*. Harmondsworth: Penguin.

Freire, P. (1973) *Education for Critical Consciousness*. New York: Seabury.

French, J. and Adams, L. (1996) 'From analysis to synthesis: models of health education', *Health Education Journal*, 45 (2): 71–4.

Friends of the Earth (1998) *Poisoning Our Children: The Dangers of Exposure to Untested and Toxic Chemicals*. London: Friends of the Earth.

Friends of the Earth (2001) *Pollution and Poverty: Breaking the Link*. London: Friends of the Earth.

Friends of the Earth Scotland (1992) *Come Clean*. Edinburgh: Friends of the Earth Scotland/Scottish Consumer Council.

Fukuyama, F. (1995) *Trust: The Social Virtues and the Creation of Prosperity*. London: Penguin Books.

Gallup (1995). *Financial Times Exporter*, Summer, p 4.

Garnett, T. (1996) *Growing Food in Cities*. London: National Food Alliance.

Gilchrist, A. (2000) 'The well-connected community: networking to the "edge of chaos"', *Community Development Journal*, 35 (3): 264–75.

Gillies, P. (1998) 'The effectiveness of alliances and partnerships for health promotion', *Health Promotion International*, 13: 1–21.

Gillies, P., Tolley, K. and Wolstenholme, J. (1996) 'Is AIDS a disease of poverty?', *AIDS Care*, 8 (3): 351–63.

Ginnety, P. (2001) *Tales from the Field of Community Development and Health*. Newry: Community Development and Health Network NI.

Ginnety, P., Kelly, K. and Black, M. (1985) *Moyard: A Health Profile. Report of the Health Needs of the Area*. Eastern Health And Social Services Board.

Gowdy, C. (1999) 'Tackling health inequalities: Inequalities in Health conference report', *Journal of Health Promotion for NI*, Issue 6, March: 4–6.

Gowman, N. (1999) *Healthy Neighbourhoods*. London: King's Fund (Public Health Series).

Grace, V. M. (1991) 'The marketing of empowerment and the construction of the health consumer: a critique of health promotion', *International Journal of Health Services*, 21 (2), 329–43.

Great Britain Parliament (1946) National Health Service Act 1946. London: HMSO.

Greater Glasgow Health Board (1994) *Report of the Women's Health Fair*. Glasgow: GGHB.

Greater Glasgow Health Board (2000) *Health Improvement Programme 2000–2005*. Glasgow: GGHB.

Greater Glasgow Health Board, Health Promotion Department (1999) *Women Talking About . . .* Glasgow: GGHB.

Green, G. et al. (1998) *SRB1 and Urban Evaluation: Baseline Report*. Sheffield: Joint Institute for Social and Economic Regeneration.

Grossman, R. and Scala, K. (1993) *Health promotion and organisational development – Development settings for health*. European Health Promotion Series No. 2, WHO/Europe, IFF (eds.), Vienna.

Guha, R. and Martinez-Alier, J. (1997) *Varieties of Environmentalism: Essays North & South*. London: Earthscan.

Hair, S. (ed.) (1994) *Glasgow's Health: Women Count*. Glasgow: Glasgow Healthy City Project.

Hakim, C. (1982) 'The social consequences of high unemployment', *Journal of Social Policy*, 11 (4): 433–67.

Halliday, M. (1994) 'Health For All briefings', *UK Health For All Resource Pack*. Liverpool: UK Health For All Network.

Hamer, L. and Ross, A. (2000) *Partnerships for Health: Policies, Principles and Practice*. Liverpool: UK Health For All Network.

Hansard (1997), 15 May, Columns 261–2, Norwich: The Stationery Office.

Harrison, P. (1983) *Inside the Inner City*. London: Penguin.

Harrison, S. (1991) 'From here to perversity', *Health Matters*, (7): 6.

Harrison, S. (2001) 'Right a bit more', *Health Matters* (44): 5–7.

Harrison, S. and Lachmann, P.J. (1996) *Towards a High Trust NHS: Proposals for Minimally Invasive Reform*. London: Institute for Public Policy Research.

Hart, J.T. (1971) 'The inverse care law', *The Lancet*, i: 405–503.

Hayward, T. (2000) 'Constitutional environmental rights: a case for political analysis', *Political Studies*, 48 (July): 558–72.

Healthy Sheffield (1993) *Community Development and Health: The Way Forward*. Sheffield: Healthy Sheffield Support Team.

Hepworth, J. (1997) 'Evaluation in health outcomes research: linking theories, methodologies and practice in health promotion', *Health Promotion International*, 12 (3): 199–210.

Herzmark, G. (1997) *Sheffield Figures: Sheffield – Gowing Together 1996 Statistical Digest*. Sheffield: Sheffield City Liaison Group.

Higgins, D. et al. (1996) *Social Capital Among Community Volunteers: The Relationship to Community Level HIV Prevention Programmes*. Abstract No. WED 3786. XI International Conference on AIDS. 2:189.

Higgins, J. (1978) *The Poverty Business: Britain and America*. Oxford: Basil Blackwell and Martin Robertson.

Hills, J. (1995) *Joseph Rowntree Foundation Inquiry into Income and Wealth*. York: Joseph Rowntree Foundation.

Hills, J. (1998) *Thatcherism, New Labour and the Welfare State*. CASE paper 13, London: London School of Economics.

Himmelstein, D.U. and Woolhandler, S. (1986) 'Cost without benefit: administrative waste in U.S. health care', *New England Journal of Medicine*, 311 (7): 441–5.

Hogg, C. (1999) *Patients, Power and Politics: From Patients to Citizens*. London: Sage Publications.

Hsieh, C.C. and Pugh, M.D. (1993) 'Poverty, income inequality and violent crime: a meta analysis of recent aggregate data studies', *Criminal Justice Review*, 18: 182–202.

Hunt, S.M. (1994) 'Cold hearts and coronaries', *Health Matters*, 19: 17.

Hunter, D.J. (1998) 'Notes of a discussion on social capital and its value to public health', unpublished Association for Public Health and Nexus, August 8.

Hunter, J. (1994) *A Dance Called America: The Scottish Highlands, the United States and Canada*. Edinburgh: Mainstream.

Hutton, W. (2000) *New Life for Health: The Commission on the NHS*. London: Vintage.

Ife, J. (1995) 'Community development: creating community alternatives', *Vision, Analysis and Practice*. Melbourne: Longman: 12–14.

Iliffe, S. and Munro, J. (1993) 'General practitioners and incentives', *British Medical Journal*, 307: 1156–7.

Jackson, C. et al. (1994) 'The capacity-building approach to intervention and maintenance implemented by the Stanford Five-City Project', *Health Education Research*, 9: 385–96.

Jacobs, M. (1999) *Environmental Modernisation*. London: Fabian Society.

James, E. (1970) *America Against Poverty*. London: Routledge and Kegan Paul.

Jeffs, T. and Smith, M.K. (1999) 'Informal education and health promotion', in E.R. Perkins, I. Simnett and L. Wright (eds) *Evidence-based Health Promotion*. Chichester: Wiley.

Jenkins, T. (1994) *Working Future?* London: Friends of the Earth.

Jenkinson, J., Layte, R., Coulter, A. and Wright, L. (1996) 'Evidence for the sensitivity of the SF-36 health status measure to inequalities in health: results from the Oxford healthy lifestyles survey', *Journal of Epidemiology and Community Health*, 50 (3): 377–80.

Jewkes, R. and Murcott, A. (1996) 'Meanings of community', *Social Science and Medicine* 43 (4): 555–63.

Jones, J. (undated, post-1994) *Private Troubles and Public Issues: A Community Development Approach to Health*. Edinburgh: Community Learning Scotland.

Jones, L. (1997) 'Health promotion and public policy', in L. Jones and M. Sidell (eds) *The Challenge of Promoting Health: Exploration and Action*. Buckingham: The Open University.

Jordan, B. (1998) *The New Politics of Welfare*. London: Sage Publications.

Judge, K. (2000) 'Testing evaluation to the limits: the case of English Health Action Zones', *Journal of Health Services Research and Policy*, 5 (1): 3–5.

Judge, K. et al. (1999a) *Health Action Zones: Learning to Make a Difference*. London: Report to Department of Health (June).

Judge, K. et al. (1999b) *National HAZ Evaluation Report*, Glasgow: University of Glasgow.

Judge, K. et al. (2000) *National HAZ Evaluation Report*. Glasgow: University of Glasgow Press.

Kawachi, I. et al. (1996) 'A prospective study of social networks in relation to total mortality and cardiovascular disease in men in the USA', *Journal of Epidemiology and Community Health*, 50: 245–51.

Kawachi, I., Kennedy, B.P., Lochner, K. and Prothrow-Stith, D. (1997) 'Social capital, income inequality and mortality', *American Journal of Public Health*, 87: 1491–8.

Kawachi, I., Kennedy, B.B. and Wilkinson, R.G. (1999) 'Crime, social disorganisation and relative deprivation', *Social Science and Medicine*, 48 (6): 719–31.

Kelly, M. and Charlton, B. (1995) 'The modern and the post-modern in health promotion', in R. Bunton, S. Nettleton and R. Burrows (eds) *The Sociology of Health Promotion: Critical Analysis of Consumption, Lifestyle and Risk*. London: Routledge.

Kemmis, S. (1981) *The Professional Development of Teachers through Involvement in Action Research Projects*. Adelaide: Deakin UP.

Kennedy, A. (1999) 'CDHN evaluation 1999', unpublished report, Celtic Connections.

Klein, N. (2000) *No Logo*. London: Flamingo.

Knight, J. (1997) 'The nutrition garden project', *The Cultivar* (Newsletter of the Center for Agroecology and Sustainable Food Systems, University of California, Santa Cruz) Winter.

Labonte, R. (1993) 'Community development and partnerships', *Canadian Journal of Public Health*, 84 (4): 237–340.

Labonte, R. (1995) *Health Promotion and Empowerment: Practice Frameworks*. Toronto: Centre for Health Promotion, University of Toronto.

Labonte, R. (1998) *A Community Development Approach to Health Promotion: A Background Paper on Practice Tensions, Strategic Models and Accountability Requirements for Health Authority Work on the Broad Determinants of Health*. Edinburgh: Health Education Board for Scotland and the Research Unit in Health and Behavioural Change, University of Edinburgh.

Labonte, R. (1999) 'Health promotion in the near future: remembrances of activism past', *Health Education Journal*, 58 (4): 365–77.

Lalonde, M. (1974) *A New Perspective on the Health of Canadians*. Ottawa: Health and Welfare Canada.

Lang, T. (1999) 'Local sustainability in a sea of globalisation? The case of food policy', in M. Kenny and J. Meadowcroft (eds) *Planning Sustainability*. London: Routledge.

Lang, T. and Caraher, M. (1998) 'Food poverty and shopping deserts: What are the implications for health promotion policy and practice?' *Health Education Journal*, 58 (3): 202–11.

Lang, T., Caraher, M., Dixon, P. and Carr-Hill, R. (1999) *Cooking Skills and Health: Inequalities in Health*. London: Health Education Authority.

Laughlin, S. (1998) 'From theory to practice: the Glasgow experience', in L. Doyal (ed.) *Women and Health Services*. Buckingham: Open University Press.

Laughlin, S. and Black, D. (eds) (1995) *Poverty and Health Tools for Change: Ideas, Analysis, Information, Action*. Birmingham: Public Health Alliance.

Leather, S. (1996) *The Making of Modern Malnutrition: The Caroline Walker Trust Lecture*. London: The Caroline Walker Trust.

Leff, S. (1953) *Social Medicine*. London: Routledge.

Lewis, J. (1986) *What Price Community Medicine? The Philosophy, Practice and Politics of Public Health since 1919*. Brighton: Harvester/Wheatsheaf.

Lewis, J. (1991) 'The origin and development of public health in the UK', in W.W. Holland, R. Detels and G. Knox (eds) *Oxford Textbook of Public Health*. Oxford: Oxford Medical Publications.

Lewis, S. (1999) *Beyond the Chemical Century: Restoring Human Rights and Preserving the Fabric of Life: A Report to Commemorate the 15th Anniversary of the Bhopal Disaster*. Massachusetts: Environmental Health Fund/Strategic Counsel on Corporate Accountability.

Lewis, S. and Henkels, D. (1998) 'Good neighbor agreements: a tool for environmental and social justice', in C. Williams (ed.) *Environmental Victims*. London: Earthscan.

LGA (1998a) *Regeneration and Health Audit*. London: Local Government Association.

LGA (1998b) *New Commitment to Regeneration: Working Together to Improve Our Communities*. London: Local Government Association.

LGA (2000a) 'Co-ordination of area based initiatives', unpublished working paper, London: LGA.

LGA (2000b) *Supporting the Action Zones: Early Messages, Future Plans*. London: LGA.

Lindholm, L. and Rosén, M. (2000) 'What is the "golden standard" for assessing population-based interventions? – problems of dilution bias', *Journal of Epidemiology and Community Health*, 54 (8): 617–22.

Lister-Sharp, D., Chapman, S., Stewart-Brown, S. and Sowden, A. (1999) 'Health promoting schools and health promotion in schools: two systematic reviews', *Health Technology Assessment*, 3 (22).

Littlewood, J. and Tinker, A. (1981) *Families in Flats*. London: Department of the Environment.

Littman, T. (1999) *Evaluating Transportation Equity*. At: http://www.vtpi.org/equity.htm

Logue, H. (1991) *Community Development in Northern Ireland: Perspectives for the Future*. Belfast: Community Development Review Group.

Lowry, S. (1990) 'Housing and health: families and flats', *BMJ*, 300: 245–7.

Lowry, S. (1991) *Housing and Health*. London: British Medical Journal.

Lupton, D. (1994) 'Consumerism, commodity, culture and health promotion', *Health Promotion International*, 9 (2): 111–18.

Lupton, D. (1996) *Food, the Body and Self*. London: Sage.

MacDonald, T. (1997) 'Holism and reductionism - their role in mediating health promotion and biomedicine', in *Report on the 7th National Health Promotion Managers Conference*. Carlisle: North Cumbria Health Development Unit.

MacKay, F. and Bilton, K. (2000) *Learning From Experience: Lessons In Mainstreaming Equal Opportunities*. Edinburgh: University of Edinburgh, The Governance of Scotland Forum.

Mackenbach, J.P. and Droomers, M. (1999) *Interventions and Policies to Reduce Socio-economic Inequalities in Health: Proceedings of the Third Workshop on Interventions and Policies to Reduce Socio-economic Inequalities in Health*. Rotterdam: Department of Public Health, Erasmus University.

Macleod, M., Graham, G., Johnston, M., Dibben, C. and Briscoe, S. (1999) 'A comparison a day keeps the doctor away . . . or does it?', *Health Variations*, (5): 10–11.

MAFF (1997) *National Food Survey 1996*. London: HMSO.

Maltby, S.E. (1918) *Manchester and the Movement for National Elementary Education*. Manchester: Manchester University Press.

Marmot, M.G. and McDowell, M.E. (1986) 'Mortality decline and widening social inequalities', *The Lancet* 2: 274–6.

Matthews, P. (1994) *Watered Down: Why the Law is Failing to Protect Scotland's Water*. Edinburgh: Friends of the Earth Scotland.

Mayo, M. (1997) 'Partnerships for regeneration and community development: some opportunities, challenges and constraints', *Critical Social Policy*, 17: 3–26.

Mayo, P. (1999) *Gramsci, Freire and Adult Education: Possibilities for Transformative Action*. London: Zed Books.

McBride, G. (1999) 'Scottish applications of environmental justice', unpublished thesis, University of Edinburgh.

McGlone, P., Dobson, B., Dowler, E. and Nelson, M. (1999). *Food Projects and How They Work*. York: York Publishing for the Joseph Rowntree Foundation.

McKay, S. and Rowlingson, K. (1999) *Social Security in Britain*. Basingstoke: Macmillan.

McKeown, T. (1979) *The Role of Medicine: Dream, Mirage or Nemesis?* Oxford: Basil Blackwell.

McKnight, J.L. (1987) 'Regenerating community', *Social Policy*, 18: 54–8.

McLaren, D., Bullock S. and Yousuf, N. (1998) *Tomorrow's World: Britain's Share in a Sustainable Future*. London: Earthscan.

McLaren, P. (1995) *Critical Pedagogy and Predatory Culture*. London: Routledge.

McQueen, D. (1989) 'Thoughts on the ideological origins of Health Promotion', *Health Promotion*, 4 (4): 339–42.

Melucci, A. (1985) 'The symbolic challenge of contemporary movements', *Social Research*, 52 (4): 789–816.

Mercer, G. and Barnes, C. (2000) 'Disability: from medical needs to social rights', in P. Tovey (ed.) *Contemporary Primary Care: The Challenges of Change*. Buckingham: Open University Press.

Milburn, A. (2000) 'Health and economics', Speech at the London School of Economics, 8 May.

Mitchell, R., Dorling, D. and Shaw, M. (2000) *Inequalities in Life and Death*. Bristol: Policy Press.

Moffatt, S., White, M., Stacey, R., Hudson, E. and Downey, D. (1999) *'If we had not got referred and got the advice, I don't know where we'd be, it doesn't bear thinking about.' The Impact of Welfare Advice Provided in General Practice. A Qualitative Study*, Newcastle: Dept of Epidemiology and Public Health and Dept of Primary Health Care, University of Newcastle upon Tyne.

Moore, J. (1989) 'The end of the line for poverty', speech to Greater London Area Conservative Party, 11 May.

Morgan, G. (1986) *Images of Organisation*. London: Sage Publications.

MORI (1996) *Annual Business and the Environment Survey, Summer 1996*. London: MORI.

Moser, C. (1996) *Confronting Crisis*. Monogram Series 3. Washington DC: World Bank.

Munro, J. and Iliffe S. (1997) *Healthy Choices: Future Options for the NHS*. London: Lawrence and Wishart.

Murcott, A. (1999) 'The nation's diet and the Policy Contexts', in J. Germov and L. Williams (eds) *A Sociology of Food and Nutrition: The Social Appetite*. Victoria, Australia: Oxford University Press, pp. 135–48.

NACAB (1998) *CAB Certificate in Generalist Advice Work – Understanding the Advice Process: Part 1 Aims and Overview of the Process*. London: NACAB.

Naidoo, J. and Wills, J. (eds) (2001) *Health Studies: An Introduction*. Basingstoke: Palgrave.

Newman, G. (1939) *The Building of a Nation's Health*. London: Macmillan.

Newsholme, A. (1936) *The Last Thirty Years of Public Health*. London: Allen and Unwin.

NHS Executive (1999) *Primary Care Medical Services (PMS) Pilots*. http://www.doh.gov.uk/pricare/pca.htm (accessed 9 March 2000).

NHS Management Executive (1992) *Local Voices: The Views of Local People in Purchasing for Health*. London: The Stationery Office.

Nichter, M. (1984) 'Project community diagnosis: participatory research as a first step toward community involvement in primary health care', *Social Science and Medicine*, 19 (3): 237–52.

NICVA (1998) 'The state of the sector', *NI Voluntary Sector Almanac*. Belfast: Northern Ireland Council for Voluntary Action.

Oakley, A., Brannen, J. and Dodd, K. (1992) 'Young people, gender and smoking in the United Kingdom', *Health Promotion International*, 7 (2): 75–88.

O'Brien, M. (2000) *Making Better Environmental Decisions: An Alternative to Risk Assessment*. Cambridge, MA: MIT Press.

O'Donnell, T. and Gray, G. (1993) *The Health Promoting College*. London: Health Education Authority.

OECD (1981) *Food Policy*. Paris: Organisation for Economic Co-operation and Development.

Office for National Statistics (1999) *Labour Force Survey 1998/99*. Norwich: The Stationery Office.

Oladepo, O. et al. (1991) 'The value of participatory needs assessment: in-service training in health education for child survival in Africa', *Hygiene*, 10: 40–4.

ONS (1999) *Health Statistics – Summer*. London: Office for National Statistics.

Page, D. (1994) *Developing Communities*. Teddington: Sutton Hastoe Housing Association.

Paris, J.A.G. and Player, D. (1993) 'Citizens advice in general practice', *BMJ*, 306: 1518–20.

Parkinson, M.H. (1995) 'Urban policy 1970–1995: programmes, priorities and partners', paper commissioned by the Department of the Environment for its 25th Anniversary Colloquium.

Parsons, C. (1999) *Education, Exclusion and Citizenship*. London: Routledge.

Paxton, A. (1994) *The Food Miles Report*. London: Sustainable Agriculture, Food and Environment (SAFE) Alliance.

Permanent People's Tribunal on Industrial Hazards and Human Rights (1998) 'Charter of rights against industrial hazards', in C. Williams (ed.) *Environmental Victims*. London: Earthscan.

Petersen, A. (1996) 'Risk and the regulated self: the discourse of health promotion as politics of uncertainty', in A. Petersen and D. Lupton (1996) *The New Public Health: Health and Self in an Age of Risk*. London: Sage Publications.

Petersen, A. and Lupton, D. (1996) *The New Public Health*. London: Sage Publications.

Phillips, N.A. (2000). *The BSE Inquiry: Vol. 1: Findings and Conclusions*. Norwich: The Stationery Office.

PIU, Cabinet Office (2000a) *Wiring it Up: Whitehall's Management of Cross-cutting Policies and Services*. London: The Stationery Office.

PIU, Cabinet Office (February 2000b). *Reaching Out: the Role of Central Government at Regional and Local Level*. London: The Stationery Office.

Poland, B.D. (1996) 'Knowledge development and evaluation in, of and for Healthy Communities Initiatives. Part 1: guiding principles', *Health Promotion International*, 11 (3): 237–47.

Pollock, A.M., Dunnigan, M.G., Gaffney, D., Price, D. and Shaoul, J. (1999) 'Planning the "new" NHS: downsizing for the 21st century', *British Medical Journal*, 319: 179–84.

Pollock, A.M., Player, S. and Godden, S. (2001) 'How private finance is moving primary care into corporate ownership', *British Medical Journal*, 322: 960–3.

Pollock, A.M. and Price, D. (2000) 'Rewriting the Regulations: how the World Trade Organisation could accelerate privatisation in healthcare systems', *Lancet* 356: 1995–2000.

Powell, M. (1999) 'New Labour and the third way in the British NHS', *International Journal of Health Services*, 29 (2): 353–70.

Pratt, J., Gordon, P. and Plamping, D. (1999) *Working Whole Systems*. London: King's Fund.

Prendergrast, M. (1993) *For God, Country and Coca-Cola*. London: Phoenix.

Price, D., Pollock, A.M. and Shaoul, J. (1999) 'How the World Trade Organisation is shaping domestic policies in health care', *The Lancet*, 354: 1889–91.

Priestley, M. (1999) *Disability Politics and Community Care*. London: Jessica Kingsley.

Public Health Alliance (1988) *Charter for Public Health*. Birmingham: PHA.

Public Health Alliance (1991) *Health on the Move: Policies for Health Promoting Transport – Policy Statement of the Transport and Health Study Group*. Birmingham: PHA.

Putnam, R.D. (1995) 'Bowling alone: America's declining social capital', *Journal of Democracy*, 16: 65–78.

Putnam, R.D., Leonardi, R. and Nanetti, R.Y. (1993) *Making Democracy Work: Civic Traditions in Modern Italy*, Princeton. NJ: Princeton University Press.

Redclift, M. (1984) *Development and the Environmental Crisis: Red or Green Alternatives?* London: Methuen.

Rees, W.D. and Lutkins, S.G. (1967) 'Mortality of bereavement', *British Medical Journal*, 4:13–16.

Research Unit, Sandwell MBC (1999) *Sandwell Trends*. Warley, Sandwell Metropolitan Borough Council.

Reynolds, D., Hopkins, D., Stoll, L. (1993) 'Linking school effectiveness knowledge and school improvement practice: towards a synergy', *School Effectiveness and School Improvement*, 4 (1): 37–58.

Richardson, A. (1999) *Sheffield and Electoral Wards Trends 1981 to 1996 for Selected Causes of Death including Our Healthier Nation Topics*. Sheffield: Sheffield Health.

Rissel, C. (1994) 'Empowerment: the holy grail of health promotion?', *Health Promotion International*, 9 (1): 39–44.

Ritzer, G. (2000) *The McDonaldisation of Society*. The Millennium Edition. Thousand Oaks, CA: Pine Forge Press.

Robson, B. (1988) *Those Inner Cities*. Oxford: Oxford University Press.

Robson, B., Parkinson, M., Bradford, M., Deas, I., Hall, E., Evans, R., Garside, P., Harding, A. and Robinson, F. (1994) *Assessing the Impact of Urban Policy*. Department of the Environment Inner Cities Research Programme, London: HMSO.

Romme, M. and Escher, S. (1993) *Accepting Voices*. London: MIND.

Rothman, J. (1979) 'Three models of community organisation practice', in F.M. Cox, J.L. Erlich, J. Rothman and J.E. Tropman (eds) *Strategies of Community Organisation: A Book of Readings*. Itasca, IL: Peacock.

Rothman, J. (1996) 'The interweaving of community intervention approaches', in M. Weil (ed.) *Community Practice: Conceptual Models*. New York: Hawthorne.

Royal Commission on the National Health Service (1979) *Report*, Cmnd. 7615. London: HMSO.

Runyan, D.K. et al. (1998) 'Children who prosper in unfavourable environments: the relationship to social capital', *Pediatrics*, 101:12-18.

Russell, H. (1998) *A Place for the Community? Tyne and Wear Development Corporation's Approach to Regeneration*. Bristol: The Policy Press and Joseph Rowntree Foundation.

Russell, H. (2000) *New Commitment to Regeneration: Progress and Policy Lessons*. London: Local Government Association.

Russell, H. with Killoran, A. (2000) *Public Health and Regeneration: Making the Links*. London: Health Education Authority.

Russell, H., Dawson, J., Garside, P. and Parkinson, M. (1996) *City Challenge Interim National Evaluation*. Department of the Environment, London: The Stationery Office.

Ryle, J.A. (1948) *Changing Disciplines*. London: Oxford University Press.

SAFE Alliance (1998) *Common Agricultural Policy Fact Pack*. London: Sustain.

Sandwell Health Authority (1996) *Regenerating Health: A Challenge or a Lottery? The 8th Annual Report of the Director of Public Health*. Sandwell: Department of Public Health, Sandwell Health Authority and Borough of Sandwell.

Saunders, P. (1993) *Towards Allotments 2000: National Survey of Allotment Gardeners' Views in England and Wales*. Corby: National Society of Allotment and Leisure Gardeners.

Scandrett, E., Dunion, K. and McBride, G. (2000) 'The campaign for environmental justice in Scotland', *Local Environment*, 5 (4): 465–72.

Schön, D. (1983) *The Reflective Practitioner: How Professionals Think in Action*. London: Temple Smith.

Scottish Needs Assessment Programme (1997) *Domestic Violence*. Glasgow: Scottish Forum for Public Health Medicine.

Secretary of State for Scotland (1999) *Towards a Healthier Scotland*. Cm 4269, Norwich: The Stationery Office.

Senge, P. et al., (1999) *The Dance of Change: The Challenges of Sustaining Momentum in Learning Organisations*. London: Nicholas Brealey.

SEPA (1999) *National Waste Strategy: Scotland*. Stirling: Scottish Environment Protection Agency.

SEU (1998) *Bringing Britain Together: A National Strategy for Neighbourhood Renewal*. London: Stationery Office.

SEU (2000a) *Neighbourhood Management: A Report of Policy Action Team 4*. London: Social Exclusion Unit.

SEU (2000b) *Learning Lessons*. Report of Policy Action Team 16, London: Cabinet Office.

SEU (2000c) *National Strategy for Neighbourhood Renewal: A Framework for Consultation*. London: Cabinet Office.

Sexton, S. (2001) *Briefing 23 – Trading Health Care Away?: GATS, Public Services And Privatisation*. Sturminster Newton: The Cornerhouse.

Shakespeare, T. (1993) 'Disabled people's self-organisation: a new social movement?' *Disability, Handicap and Society*, 8 (3): 249–64.

Shaoul, J. (1996) *NHS Trusts: A Capital Way of Operating?* Working paper, Department of Accounting and Finance, Manchester: University of Manchester.

Shaw, M., Dorling, D., Gordon, D. and Davey Smith, G. (1999) *The Widening Gap: Health Inequalities and Policy in Britain*. Bristol: Policy Press.

Sheffield and Rotherham Transport and Health Group (1996) *Improving Health in Sheffield and Rotherham: The Transport Challenge – Public Consultation*. Sheffield: Healthy Sheffield.

Sheffield and Rotherham Transport and Health Group (1997) *Moving Words: Responses to the Consultation on Transport and Health in Sheffield and Rotherham*. Sheffield: Healthy Sheffield.

Sheffield City Council/Sheffield Health (1999) *Tinsley Environment and Health Audit*. Sheffield: Sheffield City Council and Sheffield Health.

Sherwood, L. and Halliday, M. (1998) 'Glasgow City Health Profile', unpublished draft, Glasgow: Healthy City Partnership.

SHSSB (2000) *Community Development and Health and Social Services: A Strategy for Public Participation, Equity and Inclusion*. Armagh: Southern Health and Social Services Board.

Sigerist, H. (1941) *Medicine and Human Welfare*. New Haven, CT: Yale University Press.

Sigerist, H. (1943) *Civilisation and Disease*. Ithaca, NY: Cornell University Press.

Simon, J. (1890) *English Sanitary Institutions*. London: Cassell.

Sinclair, S. (2000) 'The WTO: what happened in Seattle? What's next in Geneva?' *Briefing Paper Series, Trade and Investment*, 1 (2). Ottawa: The Canadian Centre for Policy Alternatives.

Skelcher, C., Weir, S. and Wilson L. (2000) *The Advance of the Quango State*. London: Local Government Information Unit.

Skinner, S. (1997) *Building Community Strengths: A Resource Book on Capacity Building*. London: Community Development Foundation.

Smithies, J. and Webster, G. (1998) *Community Involvement in Health: From Passive Recipients to Active Participants*. Aldershot: Ashgate.

Smyth, M. (1998) *Half the Battle: Understanding the Impact of the Troubles on Children and Young People. (The cost of the Troubles Study)*. Ulster: University of Ulster Magee Department of Study of Conflict.

Standing Conference on Community Development (1995) 'Organisational Viewpoints', *Community Development Journal*, 30 (2): 1–2.

Standish, M. (1995) 'A view from the tightrope: a working attempt to integrate research and evaluation with community development', in N. Bruce et al. *Research and Change in Urban Community Health*. Aldershot: Avebury.

Standish, M. and Wight, J. (1996) *Action on Poverty and Inequalities in Health*. Sheffield: Sheffield Health.

Stansfeld, S.A. (1999) 'Social support and social cohesion', in M. Marmot and R.G. Wilkinson (eds.) *Social Determinants of Health*. Oxford: Oxford University Press.

Stevens, S. (1998) 'Reflections on environmental justice: children as victims and actors', in C. Williams (ed.) *Environmental Victims*. London: Earthscan.

Stevenson, H. and Burke, M. (1991) 'Bureaucratic logic in new social movement clothing: the limits of health promotion research', *Health Promotion International*, 6: 281–9.

Stirling, A. and Mayer, S. (1999) *Rethinking Risk: A Pilot Multi-criteria Mapping of a Genetically Modified Crop in Agricultural Systems in the UK*. Brighton: University of Sussex, Science Policy Research Unit.

St Leger, L.H. (1999) 'The opportunities and effectiveness of the health promoting primary school in improving child health – a review of the claims and evidence', *Health Education Research*, 14 (1): 51–69.

Teller, M.E. (1988) *The Tuberculosis Movement: A Public Health Campaign in the Progressive Era*. Westport, CT: Greenwood Press.

Thake, S. (1995) *Staying the Course: The Role and Structure of Community Regeneration Organisations*. York: YPS/Joseph Rowntree Foundation.

Thomas, C. (1993) 'Public health strategies: comparison of the conceptual foundations of the Sheffield and British government approaches', *Health Promotion International*, 8 (4): 299–307.

Thomas, C. (1999) *Female Forms: Experiencing and Understanding Disability*. Buckingham: Open University Press.

Thornton, P. and Tozer, R. (1995) *Having a Say in Change: Older People and Community Care*. York: Joseph Rowntree Foundation.

Thornton, J. and Tromans, S. (1999) 'Human rights and environmental wrongs incorporating the European Convention on Human Rights: some thoughts on the consequences for UK Environmental Law', *Journal of Environmental Law*, 11 (1): 35–57.

Toft, M., Inman, S. and Whitty, G. (eds) (1996) *Healthy Schools are Effective Schools: A Report on the HEA 'Promoting Health in Secondary Schools' Project*. London: Health Education Authority.

Touraine, A. (2000) *Can We Live Together? Equality and Difference*. Cambridge: Polity Press.

Townsend, P. (1991) 'Living standards and health', in S. McGregor and B. Pimlott (eds) *Tackling the Inner Cities: The 1980s Reviewed, Prospects for the 1990s*. Oxford: Clarendon Press.

Townsend, P. and Bosanquet, N. (eds) (1972) *Labour and Inequality: Sixteen Fabian Essays.* London: Fabian Society.

Townsend, P. and Davidson, N. (1982) *Inequalities in Health: The Black Report,* London: Pelican Books.

Turshen, M. (1989) *The Politics of Public Health.* London: Zed Books.

UK Health For All Network (1991) *Community Participation for Health For All.* Liverpool: UKHFAN.

UK Public Health Association (1999) *Briefing on Saving Lives: the English White Paper on Public Health.* London: UKPHA.

United Nations (1992a) *Rio Declaration on Environment and Development.* New York: United Nations.

United Nations (1992b) *The Earth Summit: Agenda 21.* Rio de Janeiro: UN conference on Environment and Development.

United Nations Development Programme (1996) *Human Development Report 1996.* New York: Oxford University Press.

United Nations International Children's Fund (UNICEF) (1994) *The Urban Poor and Household Food Security: Policy and Project Lessons of How Government and the Urban Poor Attempt to Deal with Household Food Insecurity, Poor Health and Malnutrition.* New York: UNICEF.

Urban Task Force, chaired by Lord Rogers of Riverside (1999) *Towards an Urban Renaissance,* London: E & FN Spon.

Urry, J. (2000) 'Mobile sociology', *British Journal of Sociology,* 51 (1): 185–203.

Veitch, D. (1995) *An Evaluation of the Work of the Citizen's Advice Bureau with Health and Social Services in Birmingham.* Birmingham: Birmingham District CAB Ltd.

Vrijheid, M. et al. (1998) *Potential Human Health Effects of Landfill Sites.* Report to the North West Region of The Environment Agency. London: London School of Hygiene and Tropical Medicine.

Wadsworth, M. (1996) 'Family and education as determinants of health', in D. Blane et al. (eds) *Health and Social Organisation: Towards a Health Policy for the 21st Century.* London: Routledge.

Wakefield HAZ (1999) *HAZ Plan.* Wakefield: Wakefield Health Authority.

Wakefield HAZ (2000, 2001) *End of Year Reports.* Wakefield: Wakefield Health Authority.

Wakefield HAZ (2001) *Inequalities in Health: The Evidence Base.* Wakefield: Wakefield Health Authority.

Wakefield Health Authority (1998/9) *Director Of Public Health reports.* Wakefield: Wakefield Health Authority.

Wakefield Health Authority (2000) *Health Improvement Programme 1999/2000, 2000–2003.* Wakefield: Wakefield Health Authority.

Wakefield MDC (1998) *Poverty Profile.* Wakefield: Metropolitan District Council.

Wakefield MDC (1999–2001) *The New Wakefield Initiative.* Wakefield: Metropolitan District Council.

Walker, A. (1990) 'The strategy of inequality. Poverty and income distribution in Britain 1979-1989' in I. Taylor (ed.) *The Social Effects of Free Market Policies: An International Text.* Hemel Hempstead: Harvester Wheatsheaf.

Walker, D. (2000) 'An unhealthy debt', *The Guardian,* 13 June.

Wallerstein, N. and Bernstein, E. (1988) 'Empowerment education: Freire's ideas adapted to health education', *Health Education Quarterly,* 15 (4): 379–94.

Weare, K. (1992) 'The contribution of education to health promotion', in R. Bunton and G. Macdonald (eds) *Health Promotion: Disciplines and Diversity.* London: Routledge.

Webster, C. (1982) 'Healthy or hungry thirties?', *History Workshop Journal*, 13: 110–29.

Webster, C. (1988) *The Health Services since the War, I Problems of Health Care. The National Health Service before 1957*. London: HMSO.

Webster, C. (1996) *The Health Services since the War, II The Government of Health Care. The British National Health Service 1958–1979*. London: The Stationery Office.

Weisacker, E. von et al. (1997) *Factor 4: Doubling Wealth, Halving Resource Use*. London: Earthscan.

Welsh, J. and MacRae, R.J. (1998) 'Food citizenship and community food security: lessons from Toronto, Canada', *Canadian J. Development Studies*, 19 (special issue): 238–55.

Whitehead, M. (1987) *The Health Divide: Inequalities in Health in the 1980s*. London: Health Education Council.

Whitehead, M. (1995) 'Tackling inequalities: a review of policy initiatives', in M. Benzeval, K. Judge and M. Whitehead (eds) *Tackling Inequalities in Health: An Agenda for Action*. London: King's Fund.

Whitelaw, S., McKeown, K. and Williams, J. (1997) 'Global health promotion models: enlightenment or entrapment?', *Health Education Research*, 12 (4): 479–90.

Whitfield, D. (2001) *Public Services or Corporate Welfare: Rethinking the Nation State in the Global Economy*. London: Pluto Press.

WHO (1975) *Health by the People*. Geneva: World Health Organisation.

WHO (1981) *Global Strategy for Health For All by the Year 2000*. Geneva: World Health Organisation.

WHO (1985) *Targets for Health for All*. Geneva: World Health Organisation.

WHO (1986) *Ottawa Charter for Health Promotion*. Geneva: World Health Organisation.

WHO (1991a) *Global Strategies for Health For All by the Year 2000: Second Report on Monitoring Progress in Implementing Strategies for Health For All*. Geneva: World Health Organisation.

WHO (1991b) *Sundsvall Statement on Supportive Environments for Health*. Geneva: World Health Organisation.

WHO (1993) *The European Network of Health Promoting Schools: A Joint WHO-CE-CEC Project*. Copenhagen: WHO.

WHO (1998) *Declaration on Health*. adopted by the 51 World Health Assembly.

WHO (1999a) *Health 21: The Health For All Policy Framework for the WHO European Region*. Copenhagen: WHO Regional Office for Europe.

WHO (1999b) *Healthy Cities: Evaluation of Programs*, at: http://www.who.int/hpr/cities/evaluation.html

WHO (2000) *Food and Nutrition Policy: An Action Plan for the WHO European Region 2000–2005*. Copenhagen: World Health Organisation.

Wilkinson, R.G. (1996) *Unhealthy Societies: The Afflictions of Inequality*. London: Routledge.

Wilks-Heeg, S. (2000) *Mainstreaming Regeneration: A Review of Policy over the Past Thirty Years*. London: Local Government Association.

Williams, C. (1998) 'An environmental victimology', in *Environmental Victims*. London: Earthscan.

Williams, G. and Popay, J. (1994) 'Researching the people's health: dilemmas and opportunities for social scientists', in *Researching the People's Health*. London: Routledge.

Williamson, B. (1982) *Class, Culture and Community*. London: Routledge and Kegan Paul.

Winslow, C.E.A. (1952) *Man and Epidemics*. Princeton, NJ: Princeton University Press.

Women's Health Working Group (1996a) *Action for Women's Health: Making Changes Through Organisations: A Resource Pack for Workers and Organisations.* Glasgow: Glasgow Healthy City Project/WHO Euro.

Women's Health Working Group (1996b) *Women's Health Policy for Glasgow: Phase 2.* Glasgow: Glasgow Healthy City Project.

Wong, T. and Morrissey, M. (1999) *Just How Poor is Northern Ireland? A Review of the Data.* NI Anti Poverty Network.

Worcester, R.M. (1998) 'More than money', in R. Scruton (ed.) *The Good Life.* London: Demos.

World Commission on Environment and Development (1987) *Our Common Future.* Oxford, Oxford University Press.

Young, M. and Wilmott, P. (1962) *Family and Kinship in East London.* Harmondsworth: Penguin.

INDEX